EBONY & IVORY

EBONY & IVORY

An In-Depth Look at Cultural Diversity

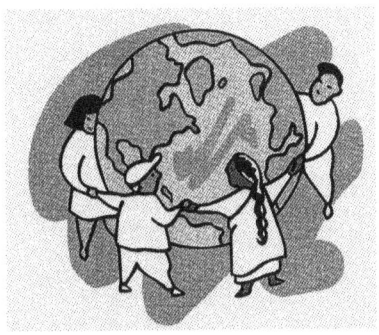

A collection of unique inspirational
& motivational stories, fables and articles
for healing BODY, MIND & SPIRIT—
and for gaining insight &
understanding for healing our Planet.

melvia miller

Writers Club Press
San Jose New York Lincoln Shanghai

EBONY & IVORY
An In-Depth Look at Cultural Diversity

Writers Club Press
an imprint of iUniverse, Inc.

For information address:
iUniverse, Inc.
5220 S. 16th St., Suite 200
Lincoln, NE 68512
www.iuniverse.com

The stories and information contained in this collection are based upon facts and truth. No promises are made of magical cures. Some names and details have been changed to protect the innocent.

ISBN: 0-595-21329-4

Printed in the United States of America

All praise and thanks are due to God for blessing me with the talent, skills, and education to compose this book.

DEDICATION:

This book is dedicated to my 2 wonderful sons, Malik and Mikal, who have been the light and delight of my life. My sons are very special people and will receive most of the benefits, proceeds and honors derived from the sales of my books. I could not have accomplished the completion of this book without my 2 sons.

~Melvia F. Miller *(author)*

THANKS:

A SPECIAL THANKS TO MY MOTHER AND FATHER for raising me. I could not have accomplished this writing project without the help, support and love of all of my many friends. I deeply appreciate all of the people who have assisted me in various ways throughout my life.

~**Melvia F. Miller** (*aka: "the Soulful Dr. Seuss*)

FOREWORD

By—Ms. Dottie Walters

Melvia Miller is remarkable! She has the vision—the dream many of us share for racial harmony, cultural diversity and peace on Earth. To write about this topic with laughter and love is brilliant.

Melvia has created this unusual book, using rhyming words and humorous stories to help break down the walls of racial and religious prejudice and cross-cultural hatred. What a wonderful idea !! She combines spiritual truths with laughter and love. I know God is smiling.

Her ideas remind me of the famous American Indian quote:

"Those who preserve their integrity remain unshaken by the storms of daily life. They do not stir like the leaves on a tree or follow the herd where it runs. In their mind remains the ideal attitude and conduct of living. This is not something given to them by others. It is their roots.

It is a strength that exists deep within them."

As I read Melvia's written words, I looked out into my garden at the blooming flowers and thought—'how well she understands God's plan for us….' All the flowers are not the same size or color or height—nor do they all bloom at the same time. God is the creator of diversity. The one golden idea that flows throughout all people was well said by Paul in his letter to the Corinthians:

"…and now remain Faith, Hope and Love…the greatest of these is LOVE."

This book is full of golden love, pressed down and over-flowing. You will love it and treasure it.

⊠⊠⊠⊠

Foreword written by **Ms. Dottie Walters,** author of *"Speak and Grow Rich"* and contributor to *"Chicken Soup for the Soul."* and also publisher of *SHARING IDEAS MAGAZINE* of Glendora, CA... *Visit her website:* **www.walters-intl.com**

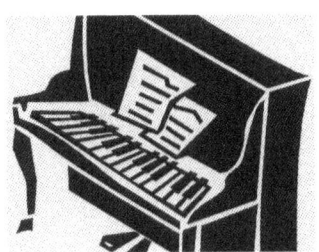

"Ebony and Ivory live together in perfect harmony…
side by side on my piano keyboard——
OH LORD, WHY CAN'T WE?

*~FROM SONG BY—*STEVIE WONDER

NOTE FROM THE AUTHOR:

CULTURAL DIVERSITY seems to be the hot topic of business conferences, college workshops, and even religious discussion groups. Our society is now made up of all types of people from a variety of ethnic groups, foreign countries, religions and traditions. Yet, America has a very poor history in coping with racial and religious differences. Many people want to hide behind **"amnesia"** *(forget slavery, forget the Japanese internment camps…forget Hitler)*—and/or want to pretend that our country has **no** problems in the area of race relations. It is a fact that the USA has had one of the worst records of racism to ever exist in the history of the world. When we all come to understand that fact—we can begin to heal our wounds. An old African proverb states:

"He who hides his disease cannot expect to be cured…."

History has many lessons from which we can all learn. In order to understand where we are today and why—we must examine the building blocks (history) that lead us to this present social situation. Thus, most of this book is based upon historical events, ordeals and facts that brought us to the place that we are in today. Many scholars and politicians have advocated that we become "color blind"—and that we ignore and abolish all traces of cultural heritage—in essence that we become a "melting pot." Well—that idea has never worked !

It is a foolish fallacy to think that people should give up their proud heritage, their history, their ancestor's culture—simply to fit into the general White society in America. It is not healthy to expect such an occurrence. Actually, we are more of a "salad bowl"—with all the ingredients *(lettuces, tomatoes, onions, croutons, cheese, herbs, spices, etc.)* joined together in the salad to create a delicious dish. Let us learn to be as we are—to be proud of the best that our culture has produced—and to learn from what history has taught us. Let African Americans celebrate their brilliance—just as much as do other groups of people.

I have written these 12 stories, fables, articles, and creative writings in the spirit of shedding more light on the prejudices and darkness that haunt us, and to help heal our wounds. Words can help us to heal. TRUTH is the LIGHT.

The "fables" contained in this book are based upon some real situations, but they are fictitious and written to give moral or other implied messages about significant issues—much like the famous Aesop did with his fables and tales.

The other stories and articles are based upon truth and actual events of history, but have been composed in a manner as to help readers get a better understanding of the problems. Above all—learn something **and enjoy the journey.**

~ **Melvia Miller,** author of *EBONY & IVORY…*
(creator of "Salad Bowl Seminars"—on the Internet)

WARNING: **Laughter and smiles may result from reading these stories.**

CONTENTS

COLLECTIBLE FABLE—#1

"New & Different Friends"

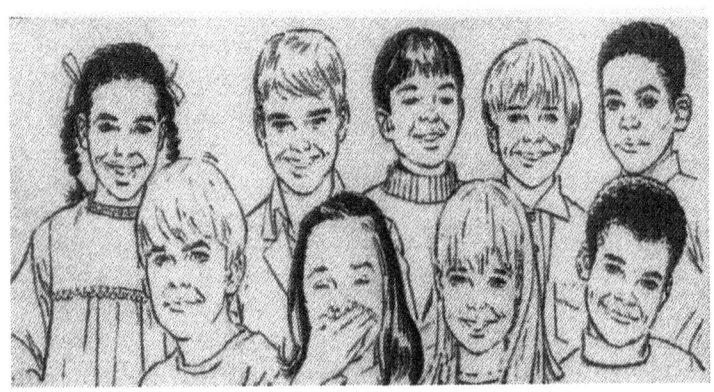

A heart-warming epic poem—
told completely in rhyme.... about how young people learn to
understand other cultures and to get along with folks of many
different ethnic groups.

By Melvia F. Miller

CHAPTER ONE

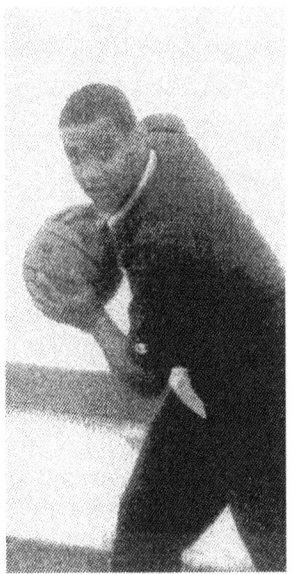

On a bright sunny day
Akbar went outside to play.
He dribbled his ball through the doorway,
Smiling all along the way....

He stopped by the steps to view
—where his buddies and friends usually sit.

He excitedly said…
"I have some news and I want to tell you about it."

"I have got something I need to say…"
Akbar told them, *"I can't shoot the hoop in a game today…*
as I came to tell you all that we will be moving away…."

"To where, " one friend asked Akbar.
Akbar replied, *"I don't know but Mama says it's far."*
We have packed all our stuff in a truck and
We will drive a long way in the car."

Akbar explained,
"My daddy's company is moving us all….
My dad is a scientist like
George Washington Carver—You may recall…
Remember—we read a book about
Benjamin Banneker and him.
My father does work like them."

A large group of buddies
Gathered around
To find out why Akbar was
Planning to leave town.

"….and my mother also had good fortune;
she may become famous soon.
My mom worked on writing really hard…
And she just won an award."

"That's real good," responded Ben.
"I guess you will be leaving soon then?"

Akbar just grinned.
"Any idea when we will see you again?"

"Her book that she wrote,"
Akbar went on....
Will soon be on sale—"
"Yes, brotha—, mo' money...mo'money!!"
—chanted Hasani.

...Akbar continued on...
"...and a check for us is coming in the mail."
"Tell us, is her book serious or funny?
—questioned Hasani.

So Akbar explained—
"It is a book of humor & history...
Her book is about strong women...
Like Harriet Tubman and Shirley Chisholm.
Mom also makes sarcastic comedy,
And also pokes fun at society's racism."

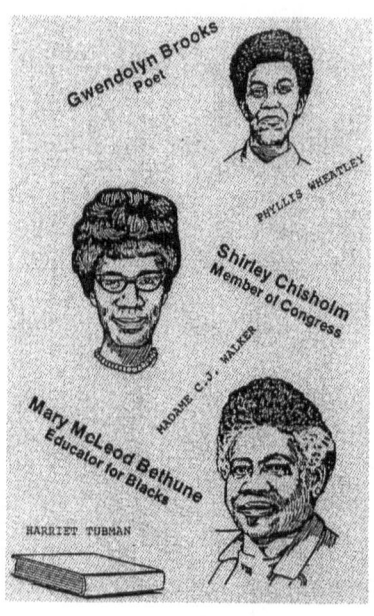

"My mom taught me
the true value of history.
She says—we all need our roots to grow
like a tree…
To become strong and free.
We should learn about our Black heroes,
Like: Frederick Douglas and Marcus Garvey
—who fought for our liberty."

"WOW!! We want to hear some parts of this book!!!
We want you to read some of what she wrote."
All the guys gathered around with their hungry looks,
And Akbar could see that he was out-voted.

Because his friends kept saying "Please…"
Akbar then opened the book to a good anecdote:

Before he started to read….
He told the guys that this story is about cultural harmony—

THE STORY:

A Caucasian (white man) mailman worked in a poor, slummish Native American Indian neighborhood—(aka: *Reservation*). He had become very friendly with many of the residents.

One day he picked up a letter from a mailbox at one of the houses. The letter was addressed and stamped to be delivered—

"TO GOD."

Well, the kind old mailman knew the kid who lived there, so he took the letter back to the Main Post Office and opened it.

The letter said—

DEAR GOD—

MY MOTHER AND I REALLY NEED YOUR HELP. SHE HAS BEEN VERY SICK AND CANNOT WORK. SOMETIMES WE

HAVE NO MONEY FOR FOOD OR THE BUS. I HAVE BEEN VERY GOOD. WOULD YOU SEND US $100???? Please.

THANK YOU.

SIGNED: **Kapone** *(Little Eagle)*

Well, the kindly old white mailman felt compassion for this boy and his mother. He arranged to take up a donation from his co-workers that day. The mailmen pooled together $50. Then the mailman put the cash in an envelope and addressed it to Kapone. The next day he delivered it to the boy's mailbox.

Several days later, this same mailman found another letter in the boy's mailbox—addressed: *"To God"*

So, the mailman took this 2nd letter back to the post office and read it aloud to all the mailmen there who had made donations.

THE 2ND LETTER SAID—

Dear God—

Thank you so much for helping me and my mother. But, God, you have to be careful about sending cash in the mail. One of these paleface mailmen stole $50 out of the money you sent us.

Signed: Little Eagle

All the guys laughed and laughed…
"this really shows how stupid racial mess can be…"
One of them shouted.."*Now that is a real gas !*"
"Your mom did a good job from what we can see."

Suddenly there was a lot of noise
Coming from Akbar's front door…
There was nothing but shock on the faces of the boys…
As they watched two men loudly roar.

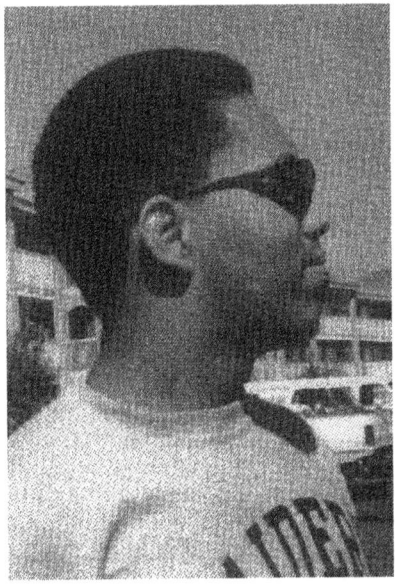

Akbar's tall daddy was one of the men,
And the other was his landlord.
These two were having a serious argument—
and neither held their harsh words.

One of Akbar's friends questioned—
"I bet you will not miss this slum?
Every week, we all know,
the landlord keeps up trouble...."
"*Yeah—and he never fixes a thing—*
he thinks we are dumb !"
And then someone added,
"*...every year the rent is doubled...*"

They could hear Akbar's dad, Ashanti, shouting—
"*Yes, we are leaving this trap.*"
And the landlord yelled,
"*Well, good—and don't come back!*
I am not worried—renting this place will be a snap."

And Ashanti responded back...
"You have never even hammered a tack..."

Akbar watched his father place proper blame....
Even though the argument was loud—
Akbar felt very excited and proud.
"*You ought to be ashamed....*"

Again, his father snapped.
"*Hey, son,* " Akbar's dad softly spoke, "Wow!!"
"*Come on home now.*
I do not want to hear any more of Opie Taylor's yap..."
"Dinner is ready!!" came a sudden shout
from the doorway.
"Well," Akbar said, "I will see you all another day."
"I'm OUT..."

He thought about how much
He would miss all that fun,
And all the fun things they had done—
They used to play out in the sun….
….they'd dunk basketballs and run.

"Do you think you will meet new friends over there?"
Ben put his arm around him and Akbar answered,
—*"I guess I will Ben Ware"*

Akbar walked toward his house and
waved goodbye with his hand…
When he could no longer see his buddies, the tears ran.
The next day, Akbar and his family
Left in a big moving van.
And again all over his face,—more tears ran.

All down the highway his mother Nubia talked as if she were a history guru…
Which caused Akbar to have dreams and
a sense of 'deja-vu.'

She read parts of her book so
they would not get bored.
Some of her work was about how black and white people are so
much alike…..
And as they rode—they laughed loud and roared.

His author mother poked fun at how people fight over equal rights……

SHE READ A SECTION ABOUT VIETNAM—

"the Vietnam War was only a time that the White Man sent the Black Man to Vietnam to fight against the Yellow Man for a country that was stolen from the Red Man in the first place.

The conversation continued in synergy—
"Dr. King lead a MARCH ON WASHINGTON
because he said the Black people live in a
'sea of poverty'
in the middle of the world's richest nation—
the so-called... LAND OF LIBERTY."

Nubia continued to read from her book so
they would not get bored.
Some of her work was about how black and white people are so
much alike.....
And as they rode—they laughed loud and roared.

Now, we all know that Black folks too are guilty
Of having their own ways of being cold and mean,
Indulging in self-hatred and low self-esteem
We have not yet learn how to live in unity."

Yes, too much BLACK-ON-BLACK crime,
And out of control GANSTA' hatred and hostility.
Dr. Martin Luther King would lose his mind,
If he could see what how blacks live in the inner cities.

Nubia read some more comedy
about Black people too....
Just for a few giggles and laughs
To make the travel time quickly pass....

YOU MIGHT BE IN A GHETTO IF—

1. If you ask someone who is standing on the corner for directions—and they cannot tell you how to get anyplace outside a 5-block radius from where you are.

2. The large neighborhood school is old, dilapidated and looks more like a run-down warehouse.

3. If you are in Church and there are at least 2 other churches like this one within walking distance.

4. If you are in a church service and a woman tells the preacher she wants to be baptized from her "NECK down"—...because she just got her hair done.

5. If you are in Church on Sunday and it is 3:15 pm and they are still preaching.

6. There is a BUILDING FUND OFFERING—but nothing new has been built in 20 years.

7. There is a tavern and drug-house within 2 blocks of the church…and each of them have more traffic than the Church does.

8. If there are several adult men standing around on corners nearby, wearing their pants drooping over their buttocks—apparently doing nothing.

As they rode toward the City border limits
They passed through a business district—high class…
Ashanti slowed way down to keep the speed limit—
Because it was no place to be caught driving fast!

SUDDENLY, there was a siren's noise;
The police forced Ashanti to stop;
Fear and anxiety drifted over the faces of the boys;
As they saw stepping out of the cop
car a big pink-faced cop.

Ashanti leaned out the window and asked,
"Did we break a law?"
"Shut up, boy!" the officer replied, *"Naw !"*
"I just saw you darkies driving suspiciously
—really acting kind of squirrel-ly!

"Is there a LAW against driving a new car around?"
Nubia spoke up and inquired…
"Naw! It ain't no law—but it is sundown
and I have to keep you darkies in my sights."

"So, you are just checking out Blacks?
Ashanti asked out of his window…
The cop answered back—
"Well—you people do crime a lot….
"Now get on out of this area real fast !"
Yelled the big pink cop.

Ashanti rolled up his window while in shock,
But they could still hear
the yells of the big red-faced cop
"MOVE ON DOWN THE ROAD AND DO NOT STOP."

Nubia responded… *"This type of police oppression*
is what caused the other recent
March on Washington
—Just ignore this fool, dear, be patient."

Akbar asked:
"Mom, do you hate all White folks—
…………*-think they are devils…?"*
She replied, *" Heavens No! Now you know some of my best friends are*
White—oh, no! But let's be honest…no sense in lying…
I look at the situation the same as the cops say about the pain of racial
profiling—
I just consider that:
WHITE FOLKS FIT THE DESCRIPTION of the ones who dished out
a lot of stealing and lying."

"Son, I look at people's actions
and how they treat me
Skin color often has a connection
But but does not always determine one's personality."

Ashanti analyzed the situation in brief—
"We just get tired of White Folks hypocrisy…
They let these foreigners from the Mid-East
come over here without any grief…
and many of them are just terrorists;
but everyone in the world tries to make
the Black people's lives hard.
Oh-my God—IS THERE JUST NO JUSTICE?"

Everyone in the car got quiet
When Ashanti yelled out….
"That is why the crowds of people shouted
"NO JUSTICE…NO PEACE"
during the Rodney King riots"…..

Ashanti responded:
"Yes and inside, this nation,
we already had a war—
in the 1860's—no need to repeat it…
It was really over whether whiteness is superior
And we know that the slaver masters were defeated."

Ashanti remarked with energy:
"You make good points, my dear wife,
American politics have not given
Black folks the good life!"
And in public education—
-folks like Dr. M. L. King had to go to jail…
Plus, we had to get Congress to pass legislation."

Ashanti added his support—
"Yeah, we had to fight just to vote…
and in 2001 the president was selected
by the Supreme Court—
avoiding counting the votes—
many Black people felt cheated due to the fact
they just over-looked the law that says
"the President must be elected."

Nubia continued read from her book so
they would not get bored.
Some of her work was about how black and white people are so
much alike…..
And as they rode—they laughed loud and roared.

CHAPTER TWO

A long while later, they finally arrived.
The new house was big with lots of trees…
The family stood in front with pride;
Akbar's daddy was very pleased.

Later, Akbar stared across the street
At some boys whom he wanted to meet.
Some of them were talking in a group;
And a few boys were shooting at the basketball hoop.

Akbar wanted to hang out,
So he walked over and gave a shout…
"HEY!!"—they all said as they stopped
playing their game….
"What's your name?"

"My name is Patricia," said a girl
who was drawing a picture on the ground.
"And this is Alberto, Carlos, Pierre and Earl….
We are just sitting around."

Akbar asked, with a smile in his brown eyes,
"Hey, I am new around here, you guys.
What is there around here to do? "

Carlos replied,
"Have fun, play basketball and some touch football—and go to
school."

Another guy said, *"They do have teams around",*
   "A guy named Henry has a team—
   may be he will choose you to play…"
"Yeah" George responded,
"Can you dribble and shoot the big round?"

"Man, our team was the basketball champion
where I lived before…" Akbar grinned.
"The crowd would roar when I dribbled
out on the floor."
"Wow!" When we see Henry, we will mention this to him."
*"OK…cool !!—DO THAT…*he grinned again.
"Yea, we will…we like to win."

Dinner is ready !!" came Nubia's sudden shout
from the doorway.
"Well, "Akbar said, *"I'll see you all another day….*
You'—all be cool…and I will see you at school."

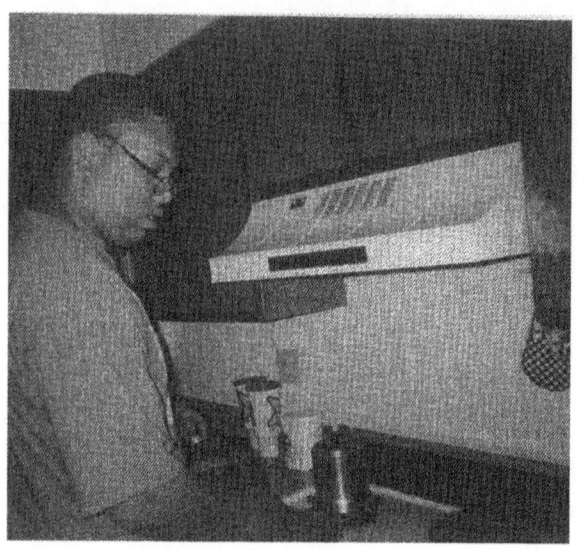

Today Akbar's daddy would serve as the chef....
He could really make good meals.
Both his mom and dad bowed their heads with words,
so the food would be blessed....

They used lots of vegetables, vitamins, herbs
and organic health foods.
Just for fun, Akbar often called his dad
"the holistic dude."

"Say....everyone....have you read this joke?"
That was Akbar's sister who spoke.
She liked any humor about the way they eat....
*"Check out this joke—it is from Mom's book
...it is really neat comedy..."*
She read the joke—

"An old man and his old wife died and went to Heaven. When they arrived, an Angel & Saint escorted them to a beautiful apartment-suite, overlooking a fabulous pond, tennis court, volley ball court, golf course, and garden. The suite was filled with all types of luxuries, including a fire-place and Jacuzzi.

The Saint told them—*"Welcome to Heaven, this will be your apartment and you can use the gardens, play the games, and just enjoy yourselves here. If you get hungry, just call room service and they will make you the best of meals."*

"Wow,"—said the old man. Then he looked at his old wrinkled wife with a mean face. She was shocked and asked him...*"What is the matter? Don't you like it??. We were good on Earth and got to Heaven."*

Then the old man scolded her—
"OF COURSE I DO. Hell, we were struggling on Earth—We could have been here 20 years ago if you had not made me eat all that vegetarian food, herbal drinks, vitamins, and soy food !!"

EVERYONE CRACKED UP and LAUGHED....
If anyone had a good humorous fable

Over the HEALTH FOOD situation, to tell at the table...
This family would wait to listen in great anticipation
Of a major session of who could laugh the fastest.

And Ali, the younger brother,
was standing there smiling

about his Mama's new book.
He was very happy about the big book deal.

He said, " *well if you all want to, we could take a vote*
On the part of her book that is your favorite fable…."
"Well, I think Mom's book is better
 than most stuff we see on Cable….
this is my favorite the one about the Indians
—to me the best one she wrote:

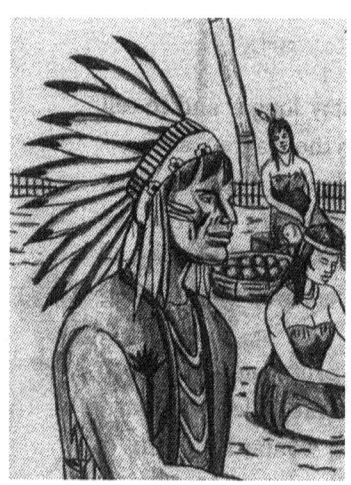

"Hoya"
It was election time and a politician decided to go out to the local
reservation and try to get the Native American vote. They were all
assembled in the Council Hall to hear the speech.

The politician had worked up to his finale,
and the crowd was getting more and more excited.
"I promise better education opportunities for Native Americans!"

The crowd went wild, shouting *"Hoya! Hoya!"*
The politician was a bit puzzled by the native word, but was encouraged by their enthusiasm.
"I promise gambling reforms to allow a Casino on the Reservation!"

"Hoya! Hoya!" cried the crowd, stomping their feet.

"I promise more social reforms and job opportunities for Native Americans!"

The crowd reached a frenzied pitch shouting—"Hoya! Hoya! Hoya!"

After the speech, the Politician was touring the Reservation, and saw a tremendous herd of cattle.

Since he was raised on a ranch, and knew a
bit about cattle, he asked the Chief if he could get closer to take a look at the cattle.

"Sure," the Chief said, *"but be careful not to step in the **hoya**."*

✳✳✳✳✳✳✳✳✳✳✳✳✳✳✳✳✳✳✳✳

Nubia's book put smiles on their faces….
they laughed loud and roared.
One would have to be a mental case
Not to enjoy these stories……

Ashanti told his family that his favorite part
Is where she wrote—

"What if slavery had been in reverse?
What if the greatest crime in history—
Black Africans had started it?
And Black folks had put Europeans in slavery first?"

THEN HE READ THIS PART:

Can you imagine a big black man with a whip—??
Beating and whippin on a white guy…yelling——

"What's yo' name, boy?"

BLACK MASTER: "What's yo' name, boy?"
WHITE SLAVE: "My name is Joseph Jones."

Pow!!! Wham!! Pow!! (sounds of whip hitting white man>)

BLACK MASTER: "What's yo' name, boy?"
—"I ast you yo' new name boy!!!"

WHITE SLAVE: " My name Joseph Johnson."

Pow!!! Wham!! Pow!! (sounds of whip hitting white man>)

BLACK MASTER: "What's yo' name, boy? I gonna cut off your foot if
you run away agin!!" I done told you your name is Kunta Zulu… "

Pow!!! Wham!! Pow!! *(sounds of whip hitting white man>)*

WHITE SLAVE: OK, OK, OK, my name is Zulu!!"

Nubia responds,
"My point is that this is a good way to calculate—
-if something is wrong or right.
Change the role of who's being violated.
This process always improves one's insight."

Soon dinner was over and done…
And the family sat around the fireplace
And they talked and had a lot of fun…
Until sleep came over all their faces.

That night Akbar slept in his own new bed.
His brothers and sisters had their own
Rooms too—just like daddy had said.
This was an order very different and new
From the times when dad's dollars were few.

The next morning was bright and sunny.
Akbar's mama said, *"Get up, get dressed*
Eat some toast and honey.
First thing today, we're going to the store."
And quick as a flash, Akbar was dressed
And waiting by the door.

Inside the store there were other boys
Playing with Nintendo and toys…
"Hi," Akbar was heard saying
to 2 boys who were playing
with some of the games and toys.

One boy asked, *"Have I seen you around here?"*
"Yes," said Akbar, *"We just moved over near the Pier."*
It so happened that they all lived quite near
And none of them had to go far.

The guys found some remote control cars
That played musical tunes;
And they saw as clown who was
Blowing up big colorful balloons.

The man blew up 2 balloons: One white and one red.
"Watch it float up high," the man said.
But the boys put their attention on the tunes
Coming from the electronics room.

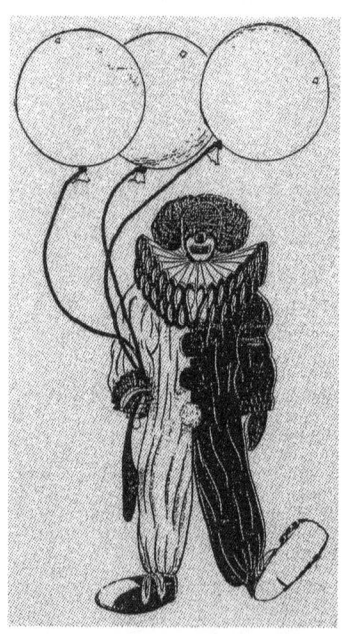

He blew up some red, white and yellow too.
He even had some that were green and blue.
Then the clown blew up a black one
And one that was brown.
They went just as high and did not come down.

While the boys watched the balloons
floating way up high,
Akbar's mother came over and told them
It was time to say GOOD-BYE.

The next day Akbar went
To Thomas Edison School—
Out in a neighborhood
Really quite beautiful.

All the students had fun in the gym;
Later his teacher gave a lesson on Pilgrims
And they watched a video
About World War Two…
And Hitler's bad treatment of the Jews.
Then to the cafeteria they had to go.

After they got home later that day,
Akbar went outside to play.
Outside he met some other boys:
Lin-Ton, Juan, Chan and Roy.

Another boy, who said his father was a car dealer,
Walked up pushing a small off-roader "4-wheeler."
All the boys excitedly asked, *"Can we get on?"*
"…let's all take turns, ride downhill and have some fun."

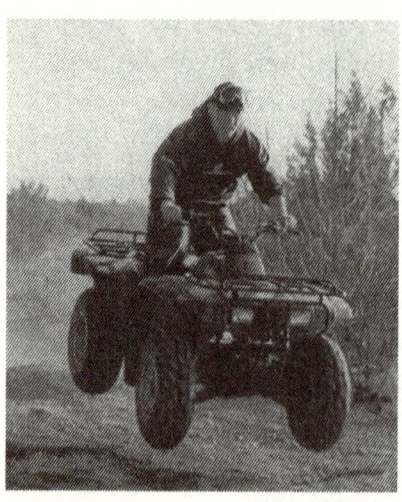

"Sure you can," said the boy....
"that is why I came...."
"Say"—said Akbar, *" I remember your name!!*
We talked a little at the store
Just before I had to go away."

"Glad you remember, " the boy replied,
but you cannot ride !!"
All the other boys—with faces of surprise—
Asked: *"Why not Henry?*
We could take turns or sit side by side."

"I thought we were going to have him on our tournament team...."
Akbar smiled a little kind greeting...
"Oh!! Is this the guy you talked about a day or 2 ago?"
Henry beamed.
George responded,
"Yeah, we thought you'd like to meet him."

"Well, he looks strange…"
I do not like his hair and his eyes…"
Well!! …Akbar had never met
Anyone like this guy.

"Now that I look at you—
I'd bet that you also play that wild style
Of jungle ball…."
In his mind Akbar thought…*"hit him in the jaw.."*
But his conscience said it was not the right thing to do…
So Akbar shouted…
"..and I bet you play that Mayberry-style ball…
not very well at all…."

Then Akbar asserted rudely,
"You do not like my eyes or hair !!!??
Guess what, Howdy Doodie,—
I do not care…"

Akbar turned around and started to run
He thought to himself,
"Is there no end to fighting racism? This is no fun.
He thought,
"There must be plenty of places to hang out and play…"

And just then he looked up and saw his daddy
With a big box in their driveway.

"Hey, Dad, what is that..? Akbar asked.
"New clothes, a bike, a bed?"
"No,—it's a video game system," his daddy said.
"We can put it together—I will be your aide.
It is your gift for getting good grades."

Soon there were kids in the yard on the patio
From everywhere
Wanting to see and play the games on video.
They forgot about the problems with Henry.

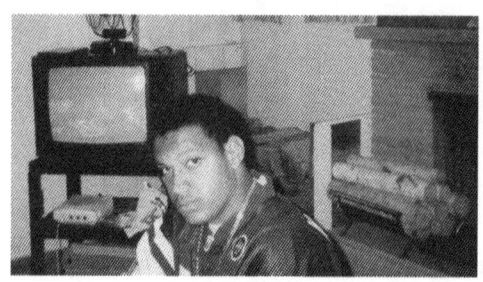

This video game was something they
expected Akbar to share….
As they stared at the game on TV…
One guy said…
"Akbar you are very lucky…"

To which Akbar replied…
"It is not LUCK—but from hard work and study…
My daddy got this new home from his work and study
And our family is riding the high tide
Because my mother and dad are also good buddies."

CHAPTER THREE

"It wasn't long before Henry
walked up the drive-way…
He could see how they all grinned,
So, of course, he wanted to play, too.

Henry asked Akbar…"*Can I come on the patio
And play with the video?*"
Akbar told him,
"*No—I don't think so…Not with eyes so blue.*"

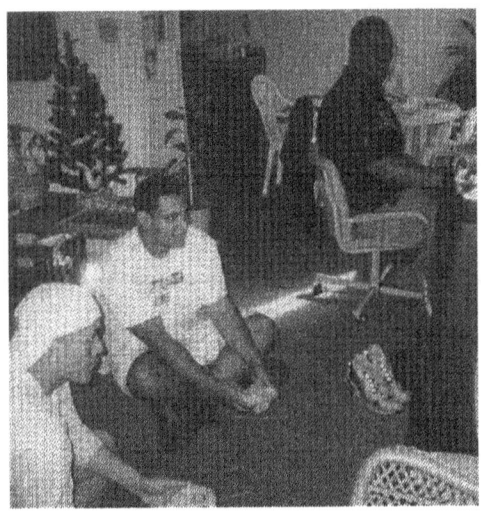

"Just what do you mean?" Henry complained.
Akbar answered him with a snarl….
"Remember what you told me about the 4-wheeler
when I remember your name?'

"Well," said Henry, *"You are just very different."*
So Akbar answered….
"who are you trying to convince?"
Lin Ton said, *" My daddy told me everyone is different."*
And then Chan spoke up and said,
"Man you are talking a lot of non-sense."

So Henry began to confess….and he sighed…
"I have never been around people who are brown."
By this time, Henry looked like he wanted to cry.
Juan responded…
"Skin color is something you cannot hide,
but my mama told me that
what counts is what is on your inside!"

Ali spoke up and said…
"My dad says—it would be a shame
If everyone looked the same."
"Yes—lord—and if we did all look alike
which ugly face would it be like?"

Then Akbar added his two-cents
"Remember the balloons we saw floating up high…?
You know, the ones that the clown had—
—no matter what color, they all reached for the sky.
This should be an example that makes sense."

Suddenly there was some loud noise;
From up the street came 2 more boys…
Carrying a huge radio and talking loud;
They also joined the patio crowd.

And he continued preaching and teaching….

As the music blasted,
The heat of the conversation lasted…
They all talked really fast,
And nobody could get a clear idea past.

Finally Akbar changed the tone and shouted….
"I like Marvin Gaye and "The O'Jays"
…. and what they had to say…
His tunes were cool in my dad's day.
His music is called old school,
But the words are still good news."

Akbar started to sing—
"….. don't they care??
What is happening to the air…?"
"Oh—mother, mother—there's far too
many of you crying….
there's too many of us dying…

He continued preaching….
"I expected that this neighborhood
would be fairly good.
I do not want to be around any gangs—
I like what old school singers sang…."

Ricardo laughed and said,
"Henry is not dangerous or violent;
He is just backward and ignorant.
He is just like a lot of Caucasians…
—that racial mess non-sense fills his head."

Akbar shouted back—
"That is what starts hate crime.
It is a known fact…
Usually a cross is burned in a short time
—it does not take a genius to now that…!!!"

"Well, let me tell you—when my family is together,"
Henry stated….
"My aunts and uncles claim that Black folks never invented any-
thing!
They talk about things like how—
white folks built this whole nation…
and how Blacks just want something for
not working—for nothing !!"

THEN AKBAR'S SISTER STEPPED OUT ON THE PATIO.

All Akbar could say was: "Uh-OOOO"
She was listening through the window…
This young girl started yelling without a *'hello…'*

"Hey,—I have a hunch
that your family is real dumb bunch….
SOMETHING FOR NOTHING!!!??
She shouted—*"Of all the nerve!!!*
Just what was the goal of the slave-masters—
Or haven't you heard the word?"

"It is quite obvious that you do not have a clue
about what is correct or true....
What was the real aim of a plantation?
Certainly not for the purpose of EDUCATION.

Plus, I bet you never heard of folks like:
BENJAMIN BANNEKER, GARRETT MORGAN, GEORGE
WASHINGTON CARVER or DR. CHARLES DREW."

Henry's response was—*"WHO ??"*
He reached up and scratched his head.
It was clear to all that he had no clue!
Henry should have shut up, but talked more instead...

"And plus you people speak English in a strange brand.
I just do not usually understand...."
To which Ali said—
"Oh really? So what? ...do we all command the language of the hill-
billy man?"

Akbar's sister Mecca yelled in to the house
For her girlfriend who was there to come out.
Majeeda was already listening to them shout... and she had
formed her face into a pout.

"Majeeda, girl, come out here"—
she yelled while giving Henry a sneer.
"...and bring Mama's little cultural bible...
there's some folks our here
that need a knowledge revival..."

Akbar then remarked...."UH, OH !!"
"Now you are in real trouble..!

Never try to degrade any Black women !
If you thought you had some problems—
They just doubled.
My sister knows her history
and will not let you win."

Majeeda preached in bliss—
"Why are you trying to cause all this stress?
—over silly ideas that are all in your head?"
"Now let me read you something about this
racial mess—
is your head DEAD?"

Ricardo chimed in….and said,
"Oh man, this is not cool.
Why do people have to fight?
Why does this prejudice thing have to last so long?"
So Akbar replied,
"The reason is there are a lot of fools,
and it seems that even when some folks are wrong,
they have to be right !!"

"Hate crimes, slavery, and even those who lynched—
all began with discrimination and stupid beliefs…
It will take a mile—if you give injustice and inch.
Mecca continued… *"Ignoring it will give no relief…"*

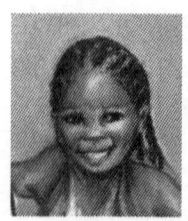

"*Hey,*" Ali suggested, "*Read some more....*"
"*Yeah,*" shouted Lin-Ton—"*your mother is very wise...*
"*OK*" replied Akbar...(*calming the loud roar*)
"*maybe laughing will help folks open their eyes.*"

SO HE SELECTED THIS PART OF HIS MOTHER'S BOOK TO
READ:

> *Scene:* A Chinese man and a Jewish man were sitting
> in a café having a coke to drink....
>
> Suddenly the Jew threw his drink into the Chinese
> man's face. The Chinese man shouted, as he wiped
> his face with a napkin...
>
> "*What the heck did you do that for?*"
>
> The Jewish man replied, "*That was for Pearl Harbor.*"
> "*You idiot !!*" yelled the Chinese man. " *Pearl Harbor
> was a long time ago—and it involved the Japanese. I
> am Chinese!—you dummy!!*"
>
> The Jewish man replied in a sarcastic tone—
> "*Japanese, Chinese, Vietnamese—ALL THE SAME
> TO ME.*"
>
> So, then the Chinese man threw his drink into the
> Jew's face.
>
> The Jew yelled,
> "*Now why the heck did you do that?!!!*"
> The Chinese responded,

"That was for the Titanic."

"THE TITANIC??? You mean that ship that sunk!!!?
Are you crazy???—Yelled the Jewish man.
" *The Titanic was a ship that was sunk by an*
Iceberg…you big dummy!!!"

The Chinese man replied with a snarl,
"*Iceberg, Steinberg, Rosenberg—*
…all the same to me…."

=================================

"Oh, my goodness…."—smiled Juan.
"Your mother is a real delight…"
The boys fell into loud laughing and giggling.
"*You see how stupid people can be*
and start a dumb fight?"
Henry was very uncomfortable and started wiggling.

As the music blasted,
The heat of the conversation lasted—
They all talked really fast,
And many new ideas came up fast….

And then another guy came named Jock,
Who was carrying a big box.
Inside was a surprise—
It was a toy replica of the
STAR SHIP ENTERPRISE.

And then Majeeda spoke:
"Man this racism problem is no joke!!
Now think about who lives on this—
Everyone is odd on the Star Ship…"

"That is why I like Star Trek and Captain Kirk…
Kirk is no Archie Bunker type jerk.
They all travel in space together—
Hearts as solid as a rock…
Not even concerned about
Those ears on Mr. Spock!!"

"Well here is some news
that will make your hair stand up on your head…"
As George talked, curiosity covered everyone's face…
"My dad said that he saw a TV show that said…
some scientists think that human
life first came from OUTER SPACE."

Majeeda could not let that easily pass by—
So she said,
"There is no doubt in my mind…
that there is something alien about this Henry guy!!
He must be from that "ZONE"—the TWILIGHT."

"Oh, wow!" Roy remarked excitedly….
"One of my teachers agrees with that too.
He told me that Star Trek and Superman
are not so far from reality…
and these theories may be right.
He had read some research—it may be true—

The first people arrived here by UFOs....
That life on Earth first came here from another galaxy."

Akbar chimed in again, getting irritated....
"In case we can agree—
Even if people have different colors or features,
We came from the same seed...
All of us were equally created.
We are all the same breed of creatures."

So he continued....

"My daddy is a scientist...
and he told me to remember this little verse:

> It is not a secret or mystery—
> The human body has the same elements
> and chemistry—as everything else in the
> universe.

My father told me that it may be difficult to comprehend...
He is studying the Egyptian Pyramids...
And he said—whether or not modern folks
Believe in aliens—
The ancient wise men certainly did."

Well, Mecca was on the offense...
And she was not one to be full of pretense—
"HEY, HENRY....Didn't you learn anything
about other races and cultures?

I bet you think every invention and deed—ranging—from science
to art to literature to agriculture—
Came from White Christians…
Because they are such a superior breed..!!??"

"And you never heard a word
about any Black or Brown person
doing anything great—no 'if' and or but'—
such as inventing a light bulb
or medicines from peanuts???
A lot of Black people did something GREAT…
Man, you are just pitiful and LATE !!!

Then Henry complained: "OK, OK, OK !!!
I know that there is a lot of wrong…
But my family taught me to think this way,
And I really do not know either
Why we all just can't get along…."

"One big reason is all this phoney propaganda
about which race is superior !"
…said Mecca.
Blacks and other people of color
have had to demand
That they NOT be treated as if they are inferior."

Majeeda began to get really deep:
"And hundreds and thousands of years ago….
Outstanding folks lived in Africa—Let me tell you all…
Black people also had heroes,

Such as King Solomon, Jesus, Cleopatra and Hannibal."
When it comes to TRUE HISTORY, most folks are sleep."

"What !!??" Henry responded in shock....
"...I have never heard about anything in Africa—
No black prophets, kings and no "Black Hannibal.
...only stories of natives walking around
in those little smocks—
throwing spears and living like cannibals."

"Now this is really deep—knee deep crap!"
"Oh my goodness...." You like to cause trouble!!"
Mecca squealed away...she snapped—
"Well, what about Fred Flintstone and Barney Rubble?
Most people know that white folks used to live in caves.
But that was another situation, time and day."

So—Henry responded, he had to speak
in self-defense....
"Well, I am no idiot—I do know some history...
and I do have some sense !"
And Mecca asked,
"Like what—??
Abraham Lincoln and John Wayne?
She snarled—
"Or are you going to tell us about Tarzan and Jane?"

Then Akbar tried to intervene—
It was becoming a bad scene....

"Do you watch TV?
If you do you will see—

floods, earthquakes, tornadoes—
terrorism and anthrax attacks—
The worst problems in this world
are not people brown like me!
Man, this planet is almost ready to blow!!"

Chan interrupted and asked....
"Do you really think so...?"
"Well, I watch the news a lot, "replied Pierre.
And George responded and giggled,
"All you need to watch is the
JERRY SPRINGER SHOW !!
You will have to agree that there
are problems in the air."

"Dig on this—at my school there was a case,
where this White kid kept getting in a Black kid's face
and making ugly remarks abut his race.
It went on and on until one day this Black kid finally broke his nose.
And take a guess who got in trouble?
As is the typical situation...the cops arrested
THE BLACK KID...." explained Paco.

George chimed in...
"This same white kid called a lot of people racial slurs...
but when someone tries to defend or retaliate,
this is the way is usually occurs...
the system comes down on the victim
who was violated."

"Well I know of a story just as bad as that…"
Paco said rather upset.

"A white guy at our school hated Mexicans…
and anything Spanish that he met.…
So he walked around the stadium…
Wearing a BORDER PATROL HAT !"

Majeeda responded…*"Now that is just cold…"*
And Akbar said…"so you see what we mean?"
Now that is just OUT OF CONTROL…
And George added in…
   "This racism stuff is really a terrible thing."

"All around the planet fighting seems
to be the normal case:
People are battling about religion and God—
Fools are shooting up our schools…
Killing over color and race…
This planet Earth has become very odd.

Then the guy with the radio said,
"Hey…cool out your heads—
listen to JAZZ, RAP and BLUES…
it is really hard to choose,
but just let the music soothe
your soul and mind—
CHILL OUT, RELAX and UNWIND !!"

"Check this out, guys," said Paco.
"…another bit of news…"
"Just as an example of our crazy planet,

I wrote a paper at school,
About how this world is full of greedy fools:

Located in the Rainforests there are natural medicines
from plants that heal what ails us.
But what do big businesses do?
They wipe out the trees and animals for wealth...
Then then sell us drugs to regain our health!!

Akbar responded, " *WORD, my latino cousin!*
"At our Temple they say there is a big reason—
for these weird storms, floods, disasters,
earthquakes, and messy seasons...."

George said, " *Yeah, man, spirituality helps us to see—*
my dad told me that human greed
and lack of respect for ECOLOGY....
have made this planet crappy.
...and Mother Nature is not at all happy.

Well, Henry jumped up and ran all the way home
And came back shortly with lemonade,
Sandwiches and cake
Which his mother had made.

"Well, I guess we can be team-mates..."
Henry proclaimed, " *Have mercy on me....*
If you give me a break... WE CAN DO THOSE GAMES?
"We can start practice this week..."

And then Paco said,
"Lame brain, that was our original aim !"

Henry gave all of the girls and guys something to eat;
And they all sat around the patio and
Enjoyed the video game and the treat.
Akbar thought it all for a while…
And later looked at Henry and
Gave him a big smile.

Henry said…*"I guess we all have a lot to learn…*
Maybe it is the young people's turn…
I mean, we are the next generation..
We will have to come up with a new way of education."

THIS HOWEVER IS NOT THE END…
IT IS JUST THE BEGINNING OF HOW THEY MADE
NEW AND DIFFERENT FRIENDS.

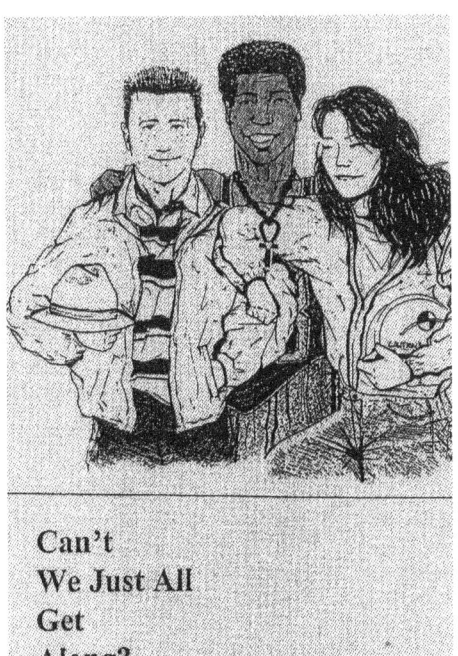

**Can't
We Just All
Get
Along?**

IN THE BEGINNING of the World...

IN THE BEGINNING...
> God created the Heavens and the Earth—
> ...out of the darkness, space, and void,
> *"The Great Spirit"*...created the Heavens and the Earth..
> —and all there is.

> The Great Spirit said,
> *"Let there be light...and there was light!"*
> And then the Great Spirit said,
> *"Let the waters be gathered and let the dry land appear"*—
> and it was so...
> There were hills & valleys, beaches, and deserts.

Next, God created vegetation *(trees, flowers, herbs, grass)* & fish, birds, and living creatures of many varieties. From the basic elements of EARTH, AIR, FIRE & WATER...God created everything that exists on all levels. God said, *"let there be beauty & truth"*—and so there was: green, blue, red, and a full spectrum of colors, which God said would work together in harmony. There were mountains and canyons and all types of sculpture on the Planet. The Creator not only created life on this Earth, but there is also life on other Planets. Each Planet and Galaxy has its on special qualities and purposes.

The work of the Sacred One was performed to perfection and took many moons to reach the time of the creation of human beings.

Next, the Sacred One created Man and Woman as help-mates to one another.

The woman was given very special qualities so that she could have children and teach them. The man was given certain other qualities so that he could be a strong protector of his family.

God created human beings originally in the land that we now know as Africa. From the darkness, God created everything. Mankind was created in God's own spiritual image….souls entered into physical bodies so that they could exist upon the physical Earth and learn from the physical plane of existence.

He decreed that these two living creatures would work together and have dominion and rule over the Creation.

Their job would be to be *"care-takers."*
And then God looked over His marvelous Creation
and said…*"it is good!"*
God created many colors of human beings.
The Great Spirit made humans in four basic colors: *Black, Red, White, & Yellow.*

And God said,
"all folks are created equal in my sight…"

And the Great Creator—the Sacred One—made special mystical herbs and plants with powers to cure, to be used for healing and curing of diseases.

He made other plants and foods for medicines and for keeping his creatures well. Mother Nature was abundant in all that the Earthly creatures would ever need to live well..including—*sunshine, air, and water.*

Millions of years ago, human society began in the place that is now known as Africa. Many ancient tribes and groups have reported that alien beings also came from the skies from other galaxies to assist the humans in developing the Earth.

Humans learned to live together in groups in order to help each other grow and gather foods and supplies. As time marched on, people learned to work together and created villages and towns, with governments.

In those wonderous days when our Earth was young and new...celestial beings winged down from other galaxies to teach arts of civilization to the unsophisticated human race—creating a Golden Age of Peace, prosperity, happiness, and harmony—which has been remembered by every major poet and romanticized in ancient scriptures and literature.

For many centuries the Earth bathed in prosperity and highly developed culture, science and arts...under the benign rule of Space Kings and Queens, who had mastered the cosmic forces and powers within the human soul.

Eventually, Africa (the land of the black & brown people) grew to be a central gathering place for the entire world at one time in history. Great temples and schools grew in the land of the dark-skinned people.

Great teachers and philosophers were teaching the people. The sciences of Herbal Medicines, and other arts emerged in Africa. Africans were smelting iron, building airplanes, and using herbal medicines—*long before the birth of Christ.*

Timbuktu was once the cradle of higher education and philosophy. The ancient Egyptians expressed their beliefs in a higher power in their writings (hieroglyphics). And in other parts of Africa, the beginning of Martial Arts *(Judo, Karate, Kung Fu, Yoga, etc.)* found their birth.

People from all around traveled to visit this great land and did trade their goods in the market places there. The ancient philosophers of

Greece and Rome all traveled to the *land of the Blacks*—Africa—to learn at the great institutes there.

Africa—*the land of the Blacks*—had become a wonderful, highly developed, spiritual land. The wonders of the Pyramids of Egypt are still a mystery to the modern world.

Ancient "super-beings" from Saturn helped build the mysterious pyramids all over the Earth. These monuments were not just for religious ritual, but also represented the secrets to eternal life.

The Pyramids are marked by writings on the walls called "hieroglyphics"—and this language is filled with spiritual symbols and signs that related the story of LIFE, THE HUMAN SOUL and CREATION. Every aspect of the structure—the tunnels, the openings, the doorways, etc.—of these Pyramids reveals the history of the planet Earth, its people and its future.

Men and women worked together, in harmony and built great societies, learned about the universal order of things, practiced spiritual arts—and the world did prosper.

Humans discovered that God had given them "free will" (choices) to think and act as they pleased.

God realized that his Creation was so vast and huge…that he knew the people would have to be spread over the face of the Earth in order to learn about and experience the beauty of the Creation.

These super-beings from other planets are those who are known in the modern world by the statues, monuments, art and carvings left by those who saw them millions of years ago.

They came in all "colors and races" from other planets—in order to inhabit the Earth. They cleared the land, procreated children and brought about human civilization.

He would eventually send a great prophet to fulfill this promise of the time of the most great peace.

THAT WILL BE THE TIME when GREAT JOY, LOVE & PEACE will emerge upon the Earth again.

That would be the time of THE MOST GREAT PEACE. So, the Great Spirit arranged that—

> White people migrate to the North to learn all aspects about AIR…..
> Black People were sent to the South to learn about WATER…..
> Red people were sent to the West to study the EARTH, and….
> the Yellow people were sent to the East to experience all they could about FIRE.

The people went forth and divided into 'tribes' and groups and separated from each other. Africans traveled across the oceans and traded with many other tribes of people.

Other groups traveled to the land known as the

"Americas"—and settled there. People learned to set up their own villages and towns.

And for a long time, there was harmony, trade, sharing, and exchanging between the various groups and tribes. Each group respected the other group.

Africans traded with the Native Americans.The Greeks traveled to Africa to study, and the Orientals also brought their wares and treasures to the open markets to trade.

If was not long until the "powers of darkness" who came from other planets also began to war against the good beings who inhabited the Earth. A major war began to rage between these forces of GOOD and EVIL.

Because some people learned about EVIL (stealing, lying, killing, etc.)…and their *"lower primitive natures"*—and chose to live by violence and greed….it became necessary for God to send humanity guidance.

But it was not long before GREED came upon the scene…..

People started to fight over religion—which Prophet was better....and some men/women became greedy, vicious, violent, cruel, selfish, and began fighting against other people who were different from their group....fighting over gold, diamonds, oil, religious beliefs, over land, over power, and over many material things.

BUT—Unfortunately, PEACE DID NOT LAST!!

THE DEVIL:

Some legends declare that many of these social deviants who caused so much trouble had actually made "pacts" with Satan (the Devil). The "powers of darkness" came from other planets to battle against the "angels of light" that had created the wonderful "Heaven on Earth."

And they became known as "the devil—or satan..."—and although at one time, these evil forces offered no threat to human civilization, Satan decided that he wanted to rule the world. So he came up with a plan to destroy anything good, constructive, positive, healthy, just, and right.

Some men became greedy and wanted to enslave other men. Tribes began to fight against other tribes for possession of certain territories. Pirates and other thieves grew in numbers.

Because of the Wars and battles that began in Heaven between the super-beings from various planets, TROUBLE, TRIBULATIONS, WARS, AND MANY BATTLES eventually descended upon the societies of the Earth.

The land known as Europe was not blessed with a good warm climate and the people there became discontent. Because of moral decay, corruption and loss of spiritual values, Europe eventually fell into *"The Dark Ages."* This was a period of time cursed by diseases, violence, and oppression.

Some of the Europeans decided to go out into the world and find their fortunes there. This was the beginning of world wide tribulation, mass slavery, and wars.

Some people became so low that they attempted to conquer and kill all the other people…simply based upon their colors and physical features.

As mankind became more advanced in using the resources of the Earth, they also became more violent, selfish and power-hungry. Even with inventions such as cars, TV, radios, computers, medical technology and other miraculous machinery—human beings continue to suffer from and wallow in a state of hostility, racism, and religious fanaticism.

God also sent many "holy prophets" to mankind to help guide them and show them the proper ways to live and be successful. He sent enlightened men such as: Moses, Jesus, Buddha, Muhammad and others.

Unfortunately, religion became a source of disagreement and disputes—rather than a resource for creating peace.

THE MOST GREAT TRIBULATION: Guns

The discovery of how to use explosives and gun-powder was the major problem that did cause the total disruption of peace on Earth. When men began to branch out and explore other lands, they found gun-powder in the Orient (the land of the Yellow People).

Although the Oriental people had only previously used their explosives for fire-works at celebrations—the Europeans found a way to utilize these powders as weapons.

Europe, which was the land of the White People, had fallen into a great depression with widespread corruption and barbaric practices flourishing. So many of the Europeans decided to leave their land and to go out to conquer the rest of the world. They traveled the world and eventually discovered how to use the explosives to make weapons. Their greed caused them to want to conquer the entire world. And with guns—they did.

The discovery of how to use iron and gun-powder to produce weapons of destruction was the mark of the beginning of a time of horrible violence, wars, and injustices.

Explorers such as Christopher Columbus and Amerigo Vespuci traveled to other lands and began to attack, rob, and kill the native peoples who already lived there. There are legends and stories that claim that these "explorers" had made agreements with the Devil....and that their actions were dictated by Satan himself.

Columbus found his way to the land known as the Americas—and even though there were many people who already inhabited this land. Christopher Columbus (and his sponsors) decided that *"they had discovered America"*—and that it belonged to them.

In the Middle East—the Arab men became so greedy that they went to Africa and fought the Black people there in order to rob them of oil, gold, diamonds and other commodities. This was the beginning of the horrible Transatlantic Slave Trade.

It was not long until the Europeans and other ethnic groups got involved in robbing the Black people of Africa. Many Europeans *(e.g. Germans, English, French, etc.)* went to African lands and wrote letters and article back home to Europeans and reported that the Black people were actually "inferior" to the Whites. This was the beginning of the horrors of RACIAL HOSTILITY.

The African Slave Trade had nothing to do with racial inferiority or the *"superiority of white people."* The slave trade was nothing but a greedy business of robbing the continent of Africa—for the sole purpose of a certain group of people to rule over the Earth and to act as ungodly dictators to the rest of humanity.

In order to perpetuate the enslavement of people, it was necessary to spread lies about the victims of slavery—to generate ideas in people's minds that the slaves were "inferior." The concept of racial inferiority was only a tool of propaganda used by the perpetrators of this horrible robbery to convince others that *to enslave the dark-skinned people was OK.*

THE INVENTION OF RACISM:

Groups of people began spreading propaganda that claimed in essence that one's skin color determines one's value:

"If you are white—you are alright.
If you are yellow—you are mellow…
If you are red—they will let you get ahead.
If you are brown—you can stick around…
But if you are Black—you have to stay back."

PROPHETS SENT TO GIVE GUIDANCE:

Out of Great Love, "The Great Spirit " sent many different prophets and messengers to the various groups of people to teach—during different time periods to teach and give spiritual guidance.

He sent—Moses, Jesus, Buddha, Muhammad, Baha'ulla, —and many others at different periods during the history of the Earth.

Moses worked for JUSTICE.
Jesus taught the great message of LOVE and ETERNAL LIFE
Muhammad taught the great message of PEACE
AND
One final PROPHET was sent to fulfill all of the Sacred One's Plans for the MOST GREAT PEACE.

...and all of them attempted to teach way-ward mankind how to live in harmony.

All of these messages from the *Bible, Quran,* and other scriptures came from the same ONE source. The Great Creator intended that there be peace upon the Earth...and that all mankind would live in harmony.

All of their spiritual messages had the same basic, essential meanings....

- WALK IN THE PATH OF GOODNESS
- THOU SHALT NOT KILL, STEAL, OR DO BAD WILL.
- LOVE ONE ANOTHER
- EAT WELL TO LIVE WELL *(health & wellness)*
- ALL FOLKS WERE CREATED EQUAL—
- ONE CREATOR CREATED CREATION—

However, many people simply used portions of the great messages to serve their own selfish goals. But in many cases, the people did not heed these holy teachers—and continued in their lowly, way-ward activities.....*FOR EXAMPLE:* Men continued to mis-treat women; Whites carried out many acts of hatred & slavery against darker races of people; and there were many wars between nations. Although lessons should have been learned from history about the horrible evils, detriment, and terrible social effects of war and slavery—many people remained in a barbaric mental state.

People separated into various religious groups and began to fight against the other religious groups—even though their prophets all came from the same SOURCE.

Each of these religious groups established leaders, and many of these leaders became fanatical in their beliefs that their way was the ONLY WAY to be *"spiritual"* or to get to God…to go to "paradise" or to die and go to "Heaven."

In fact, many of these religious zealots became so fanatical in their demands that everyone follow their particular brand of religion—that wars were started over this issue alone. War over religion has been fought more times than for any other single reason.

And this is really outrageous, pathetic and sad—since the ultimate goals of all religion or spiritual faith are: COOPERATION, BROTHER-HOOD, UNITY, WELLNESS, PROSPERITY, and PEACE.

Modern societies now suffer from many social problems that are a result of man's rejection of spiritual values and the path of the GREAT SPIRIT.

The Earth has been and remains to this day—plagued by crime, disease, hunger, slavery, riots, injustices, oppression, wars, and worse!

****

"Right is of no sex;
Truth is of no color;
God is the Father of us all
And all—we are brothers."

~Quote from FREDERICK DOUGLASS,
...(famous abolitionist & journalist)

THE SECRETS OF THE GREAT PYRAMID—

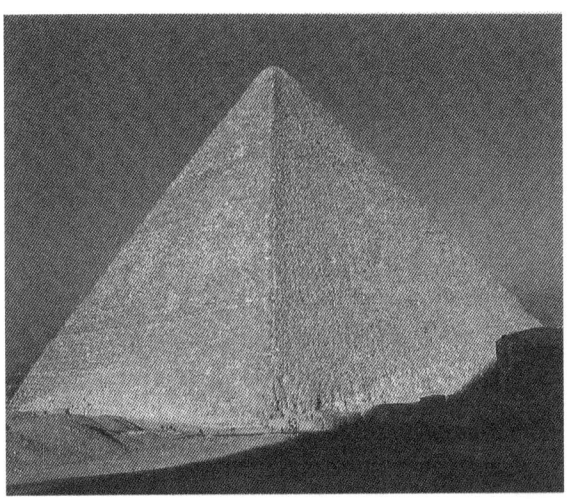

Ancient Egypt and the wonders of the ancient world, pharoahs, the Nile River, their ancient gods, and monuments have fascinated people of all backgrounds, ages, religions and cultures. Of the many ancient "wonders" of the world, there stands one monument in Egypt at the Giza Plateau, which testifies to a superior knowledge than any other old relics or buildings ever built.

The GREAT PYRAMID captures the imagination of many scientific and religious disciplines. It has been named *the "great pyramid"* because of it superior construction, design, and size.

THE GREAT PYRAMID was 454 feet tall, 760 feet long—each base, and covers an area of 13 acres of land. It contains more masonry than contained in all churches, temples and cathedrals built in Europe since the time of Christ.

Some scholars and historians have said it is "like a building let down from heaven…"

> Many historians, archeologists, religious scholars, historians, and scientists have studied the GREAT PYRAMID, which was built 2000 years before Christ was born, and have offered many theories for its purpose…..

Some of the theories included:

The Pyramid was built for—
* a landing pad for spaceships
* an observatory for astronomers
* a temple for worship
* a burial tomb
* a refuge from bad weather
* a memorial to aliens who had visited Earth

However, from more recent scientific investigations, it has been learned that the GREAT PYRAMID's dimensions, location, design and structure are so highly advanced in mathematics, geography and astronomy—that there must be a more highly significant purpose and meaning for the existence of the PYRAMID.

Scientists and astronomers have discovered that the location of the PYRAMID has a direct relationship to certain stars and galaxies in the universe.

The Pyramid is accurately aligned "true North," which is a very difficult feat for any builder to accomplish.

And the Pyramid's meridian is the natural zero meridian of the Earth. And Egypt is the geographical center of the dry land masses on Earth.

It has also been found that the tip of the PYRAMID is aligned perfectly to stars in Orion's belt…. (out in the galaxy).

Scientists and mathematicians have discovered many other remarkable and amazing characteristics of the GREAT PYRAMID, including the fact that nearly every unit of measure of its structure has a relationship to the measurements of the Earth, its distance from the sun, and measurements, such as those used to build Noah's Ark. There are some mathematical measurements that indicate the exact distance from the Pyramid to the Sun.

The mathematical relationships are so high advanced that it is obvious that whoever built this PYRAMID had a far higher degree of scientific, astronomical, and mathematical knowledge than even the modern 21st Century researchers.

Inside the PYRAMID are passage-ways, chambers, and tunnels. It has been discovered that each of these passage-ways and chambers have meanings and purposes also. The passage-ways inside the PYRAMID corroborate—symbolically—all periods in human history.

It appears that the GREAT PYRAMID is a type of holy scripture or "*Bible*"….or "spiritual message" made of stone.

THE KING'S CHAMBER is the largest room in the PYRAMID and it symbolizes "divine life."

THE Queen's chamber symbolizes an *"everlasting home"* where there will be no more sorrow, crying, pain,
death or destruction" for mankind on Earth.

THE GRAND GALLERY leads to the King's Chambers and represents the path to spirituality (GOD)...and the
righteous divine life.

THE DESCENDING PASSAGE is a wide, slippery downhill tunnel that is symbolic of the path of destruction,
immorality, sin, and death.

THE ASCENDING PASSAGE represents the promise of the good life by following the LAWS OF GOD.

Some of the mathematical relationships are astounding and beyond modern human imagination—as to how they were accomplished or conceived...because even if man did know about mathematics, the chances that men could have consolidated all this knowledge into the single expression of the construction of the GREAT PYRAMID is highly unlikely.

Now this is what is even more amazing——THE GREAT PYRAMID's structure correlates with specific events, time-periods, and significant occurences in the entire history of mankind.
FOR EXAMPLE:

a) The *Bible* describes man's life-descent...depicting man's difficulties, struggles, and ordeals.
Likewise, the Descending passage system in the PYRAMID is the long, low one that leads from the entrance to the Pit Room.

Other religions, such as Islam and Bahai Faith also speak of this same phenomena....of how life works, how to get to heaven, and similar spiritual issues.

b) According to the Bible (and other holy books)—man's first opportunity to escape "hell and death" was via following the LAW OF GOD.

Likewise....symbolically...Inside the PYRAMID is an "ascending passage"—which branches off from the "descending passage"—representing the path of salvation or chance toescape hell and death.

c) The "passage-ways" in the Pyramid symbolically bgein with Adam and Eve (first humans) and illustrates human history until the final time of a great peace.

The PAST, PRESENT, AND FUTURE of mankind's history has been divided into 3 major epochs or dispensations by scholars:

1—From the time of Adam to Noah (flood)
2—After the great flood til Christ's rise.
3—After the time of Christ....into "the Millenium"—
The time of the MOST GREAT PEACE which will last forever.

Interestingly—THE GREAT PYRAMID contains tunnels, chambers and construction that symbolize each of these time periods for human history. Many religious scholars believe that because of its amazing and profound construction, that there is alsoa spiritual significance for the existence of the GREAT PYRAMID.

These scholars advocate that the existence of this pyramid is a direct sign from the Creator of the Universe (God)....that is gives the best evidence of the existence of God.

Many of the hieroglyphic writings on the buildings also have symbolic meanings in regard to the SOUL. The ancients used the symbol of the "ankh" to represent ever-lasting life of the human soul.

The ancient Egyptians were very concerned about the"soul"—and most of their culture, writings, and ceremonies were based upon their beliefs in attaining "ever-lasting" live.

According to the PYRAMID—science, math, and religion all agree and work together in a synergistic manner. Another remarkable feature of the Pyramid is that the base is a perfect square and the 4 sides equal triangles that rise inward and upward from the base. The Pyramid is set toward true north, south, east and west....with less than 5 seconds error.

Sir Isaac Newton took the number 25, which is the number of pyramid inches in the sacred Hebrew cubit and divided the baseline of the pyramid with that number and came up with 365.242242

—which is the exact length of the solar year.

Other modern scholars, such as Dr. Naim Akbar, have studied the writings and symbols on the walls of the Pyramid and found that all of these markings have spiritual and holistic significance.

> In his book: *Light from Ancient Africa*—he clearly describes the spiritual meanings and significance of many of the symbols, writings and art on the walls of the Egyptian Pyramids. Nearly every aspect of the ancient Egyptians' lives had a connection with their spiritual beliefs.

> The significance of the GREAT PYRAMID unfolds as one studies it. It is obviously much more than just a mere stone monument used for burial.

> The wisdom, mercy, compassion, and love of God are not only written and recorded for us in scriptures, such as the Bible,

Holy Quran (and other religious books)—this knowledge is also recorded in stone scientifically—so that we can see that it was not just a random (helter-skelter) ordering of events—nor was the creation of the Earth, mankind or human history and "accident."

It is clear to those who study this GREAT PYRAMID that its purpose is far more than just to provide the tomb for and ancient pharoah or a place of burial for mummies.

THE GREAT PYRAMID appears to be a spiritually revealed message to all of us concerning the way to redemption, salvation, ETERNAL LIFE, brotherhood, harmony and peace in our lives.

———————————

COLLECTIBLE FABLE—#4

"the american dream"

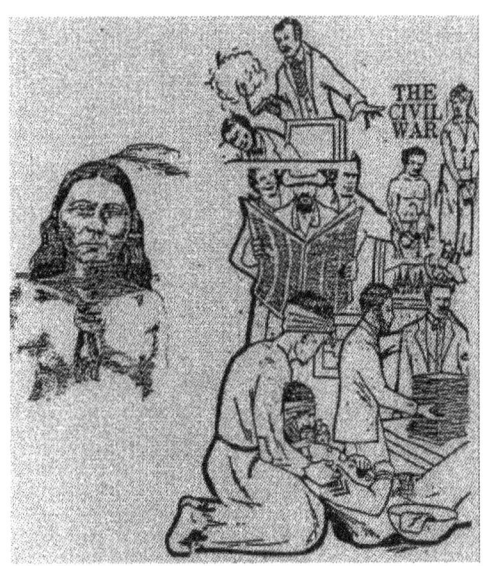

It was a beautiful, sunny day in Washington, DC. The sun reflected the shadow of the White House onto the plush green yard. A few people could be seen walking slowly near the historic capital building, but there was not much commotion on the streets at all.

In fact, it was extremely quiet—considering that Washington is usually a noisy, bustling city with tremendous traffic problems. But not today.

President George Dubyah, who had recently been selected as the new U.S. President arose from his bed and proceeded through his normal routine for the morning—exercising, washing up, and eating breakfast. He gave his usual greeting to his wife and to others as he headed down the hall to his office. The President had not been in the Oval Office more than 10 minutes when the phone rang.

It was V.P. Dick —and he was extremely upset and talking loudly—

"*George Dubyah—!!! We have been unable to locate the Secretary of State –Colonel Powell!!!*" he shouted.

The President responded, "*What are you talking about? He is usually around here someplace. Have them page him.*"

"*With all due respect, sir, we already did. We have been trying to find him all night and all morning. At first we thought it was just that he wanted some privacy for a while…but he seems to be missing,*" answered Dick.

"*Well, have you tried his home? Call his wife,*" the President replied in a problem-solving, presidential tone.

So Dick responded, "*I don't think you fully understand. We have done all of that and more. No one answers at his residence either.*"

Then the Vice President shouted…."*Oh!! Turn on your TV—Channel 5. A newsflash is on that you must hear.*"

So George Dubyah turned on the small TV in his office and watched the newscaster give a shocking report. Tim Brokow was sitting there in his usual news-reporting position talking about a major mystery that had occurred.

The news reporter stated:

"*This is a breaking news flash!! For some unknown reason, hundreds (if not thousands) of people have suddenly been reported missing. Police and sheriff offices have been bombarded with phone calls from frightened people who claim that they cannot find their friends, co-workers, and neighbors.*"

Then the reporter showed TV film footage of visions of houses and apartment buildings in neighborhoods that appeared to be abandoned and deserted—no children playing in the parks, no body walking a dog—no signs of life.

Brokow's voice intervened and said,

"Stay tuned for further updates on this huge mystery….."

George Dubyah was pacing the floor by this time. He yelled over his speaker phone to Dick—*"round up the staff and get them in here for a meeting!"*

Within 20 minutes, people were lining up to go into the Oval Office for the *President's emergency meeting.* Everyone appeared to be worried and upset.

The meeting began with George Dubyah thanking everyone for coming. He noticed that the Secretary of State Colonel Powell was not there and neither was his Security Advisor Connie.

Just as George Dubyah began to discuss the mysterious disappearance, one of his White House Interns opened the door and said,

"Excuse me sir—I know this is unusual protocol—but –it is URGENT—they told me to tell you to turn on the TV right away and watch the important developments…."

So, Dick turned on the TV so that all of them could watch it. Again Mr. Brokow was talking about more reports of missing people. This time he announced—

"This is an emergency news flash!

We have been receiving hundreds of reports about missing people this morning. Now there are new developments. We have found out that most of the mysteriously missing people are Black. Yes, millions of African-Americans—Negroes as some like to call them—seem to have disappeared from society."

Everyone in the meeting watched the news cast with amazement, shock and grief. The room fell cold and silent. They were all stunned to the point of speechlessness. The government had faced many other crises, emergencies, and even riots before—but never anything like this in the history of this great nation.

The President looked around the room at all of the pale faces and went into deep thought. This was not a problem that he ever anticipated.

Finally, someone spoke up—" *I will bet this is some kind of Democratic conspiracy !!" —A Joke!!" Yeah, they are pulling something to make the Republicans look bad....*"

Then one of the cabinet members spoke up and replied....."But *how?? How could anybody cause the disappearance of thousands or millions of Black people? It makes no logical sense.*"

Then another member of the Cabinet spoke and said..."*Well, I would not put it past them.*"

George Dubyah intervened in a commanding voices and stopped this trend in the conversation and said,

"*Let's keep our cool, now. This is obviously something very serious and not a joke from any Democrats. In fact, this is something that will require the help of our CIA and military intelligence advisors. I will call them up for reports and then we can re-convene our meeting later after we know more.*"

So everyone filed out of the Oval Office, upset but calm, and went back to their normal daily routines. George Dubyah put his secretaries to work contacting the Pentagon and other military officials.

He personally dialed one of the top Army Generals to find out what he knew. However, the General did not know much more than George Dubyah did. He calmly informed the President that a military operation to discover what caused the problem would be very difficult.

George Dubyah shouted—"*Why would it be so difficult??*"

"*Well, most of our military is Black and they are also missing...*" the General answered.

"*WHAT !!??*"—George Dubyah responded in a state of total shock.

"*Are you telling me that some of our troops are missing too?*"

The General responded, *"BINGO! Most of our troops are non-white—and they cannot be found."*

George Dubyah was now extremely upset, confused, shocked and stunned. He could not believe it. Once again he turned on the TV News. By this time there was nothing else on most channels except reports about the missing Black people.

George Dubyah tuned into ESPN *(the Sports Channel)*—thinking that there had to be some better news. But he was disappointed. There sat another news reporter on that channel who was announcing that people such as Tiger Woods, Shaq O'Neil, Michael Jordan, Scottie Pippen, Mike Tyson, and Muhammad Ali —were also missing.

"Good lord!!" he thought to himself. So he turned to another channel. This time he saw *"The 700 Club" (religious show).* However, the news was basically the same—nothing but comments about the missing people.

This time there was footage being shown from home videos that were taken by regular citizens—showing deserted neighborhoods. And they showed video of White people talking about the problem—WHITE DOCTORS, ATTORNEYS, TEACHERS, PSYCHOLOGISTS, BUSINESS OWNERS, etc.—all expressing grief over the ordeal. Most of them had lost a maid, chauffer, janitor, stock boy, cook or other workers. No African-American workers could be found.

The President's face looked like a deer in headlights.

Suddenly he had a bright idea. He thought to himself—*"I know. I will have my secretary contact the Welfare & Food Stamp Offices. I will bet that not all of these Black people are gone!*

So, he had his secretary call several Food Stamp offices to investigate this problem and then tell him if they have any reports of this kind about disappearing people. As he awaited these urgent investigative reports—he paced the floor and bit his finger nails.

It was not long before Vice President Dick contacted him again and reported the following:

"*Mr. President—we have a major problem on our hands. I just got a report from several federal prisons that all Black prisoners have disappeared !!*"

Now George Dubyah was totally upset and tears ran down his cheeks. His face turned pale as he flopped down in the big presidential chair.

He looked at Dick with red eyes and asked, "*Do you think this is some kind of civil rights protest? Maybe it has something to do with the Florida Election mess and that sloppy re-count business??*"

Dick replied, " *Well the theory is a good one—but HOW COULD THEY DO THIS?—I MEAN—how could anybody manage to make thousands of people disappear and even those from prisons?*"

The President responded—

"*Yeah—this is really something out of this world—like the Twilight Zone,*"

As Dick flopped down on the sofa in frustration—he suddenly had a brilliant thought. He jumped up and yelled—"*I KNOW…*"

"*Get that Jess Jackson and that NAACP President on the phone right away!*"

Dick looked at George Dubyah and asserted—

"*I will bet $100 bucks that they are behind this mess. It is some kind of trick or protest or something like that!!*"

"*Now that sounds logical!!*"—yelled George Dubyah with refreshed energy.

Within 5 minutes, the secretary reported to them that none of these people could be found. She also informed them that the Welfare & Food Stamp offices are reporting massive disappearances of Black people.

Now the President of the greatest country on Planet Earth was absolutely flabbergasted.

His secretary sat down to read notes to him from her investigations—

"Mr. President—the phones are being flooded with calls about missing Negroes (Black folks). White People are calling in complaining that they have no one to do the dirty work— such as cleaning up or boring factory jobs.

Many of these white people have been complaining that we may never be able to see a good football or basketball game again! And they are worried about—NO MORE "OPRAH", NO more good soul food cooking, NO "SOUL TRAIN"…no good jazz or soul music !!! Some of the white people have been very smart-alecky on the phones with our aids and complain that want you to do something about this problem!

George Dubyah responded—

"We have no answers! Our military and CIA have been unable to find out anything that would lead us to a single clue. Look, schedule a TV Press Conference and I will go on TV and explain the best I can—but only have a few reporters in the room."

Later that day, the President stood before the reporters and made his depressing report that the US Government had no idea of what had happened to millions of people of color.

After his Press conference, George Dubyah was exhausted and went home to rest. He was mentally, physically, and emotionally drained. Even so, he could not finish his dinner. He tried to sleep also, but could not. He paced the floor most of the night, despite his wife's appeals for him to come to bed.

Around midnight the phone rang loudly. It was one of the CIA agents calling to inform George Dubyah that there were now sporadic reports of other minorities group members disappearing—such as: Phillipinos, Puerto Ricans, Ecuadorians, Cubans, Haitians, Jamaicans, Mexicans,— and even some of mixed races.

George Dubyah spent the entire night pondering upon this terrible dilemna. Then the next morning he met with Dick again.

He told Dick—*"I think that I have figured this mystery out. Have someone find that Minister Louis Fakaran for me."*

Dick asked, " *I think it is pronounced—"FAR-A-KAN" ..*
...Do you think he was behind this mess?"

George Dubyah asserted—" *Well, think about it—he sponsored that*
MILLION MAN MARCH,—*then they held the* MILLION FAMILY
MARCH. *And this group publishes a newspaper called* THE FINAL
CALL.—*Now I have read that paper a few times, and in it they talk about*
some "MOTHERSHIP"—that is suppose to come and help the downtrod-
den Blacks. All this time I just thought Fakaran did not have both oars in
the water. But after analyzing it all night—maybe he is not so crazy. A lot
of people do listen to him!"

Dick asked in amazement,

"Do you mean to tell me that you read that crap?"

He told Dick—*"Well they had a lot of good information in that paper*
about Black people's achievements and contributions to the USA being
great. I learned a lot about people like— Dr. George Washington Carver,
Elijah McCoy, Jan Matzeliger, Crispus Attucks, Harriet Tubman, and
Dr. Daniel Hale Williams and so on......

Actually—that is why I read the paper—because I learned so much
about Black history. But I just never liked their stance against White peo-
ple—you know—claiming that— all White folks are Devils."

Dick replied, *"Are you telling me that you think that Minister Farakhan*
has some kind of space ship or aliens to help him make all these Black peo-
ple disappear?"

George Dubyah insisted and responded, *"Do you have a better expla-*
nation? You know we have known about flying saucers for a long time.
Heck, our Air Force has some space ships hidden out in Area 51 near Las
Vegas. We know that there are aliens who have come to this planet. So
maybe it is possible that Farakhan has pulled off a MILLION FAMILY
DISAPPEARANCE...."

Dick was stunned. He picked up the telephone and made some calls
to the FBI and CIA and issued orders to have Minister Farakhan
detained for questioning. After 3 days of an APB, broad nation-wide

search, investigations, door-to-door questioning of people—Minister Farakhan— was no place to be found.

President Bush and his staff were asked to fly to Chicago by the Chief of the FBI to visit the vacated offices of Farakhan.

What they did find there upon arrival was a pile of *newspapers—THE FINAL CALL* with an article and large bold print headlines. The newspapers stated:

===

"THE FINAL PROTEST"
To the United States Government:

We Black *(African-americans, so-called Negroes)* have been subjected to all types of inhuman and unjust treatment at the hands of White people and this government—including slavery, lynchings, church bombings, rapes, and segregation.

We are the descendents of great Kings and Queens from ancient Africa, who built the Pyramids, created martial arts, and educated the great philosophers from Greece and Rome. Our great ancestors were the originators of sciences, technology, medicines and architecture. But you ridiculed us and called us: *"jungle bunnies, spooks, coons, and jig-a-boos."*

And many of the ex-slaves that have lived in the USA have made outstanding contributions to the development of this great nation—such as people like: Dr. Martin Luther King, Mary McCleod Bethune, Jesse Owens, Benjamin Banneker, Sojourner Truth, Phyllis Wheatley, Garrett Morgan—etc.

While the rest of the nation benefited financially from our inventions—such as from the **NBA** and *Rock & Roll Music*——black people were treated a less than human.

As a race of people we have produced many great thinkers, inventors and scholars—But many our great thinkers and leaders, such as Thurgood Marshall, Marcus Garvey and WEB Dubois have never received any honors for their great leadership.

We, as a people with a common heritage, have been treated **without respect** and forced to live in poverty in a sea of wealth.

As a group of people from a common heritage, we have chronically rebelled, protested, and voiced our opposition to this ugly treatment.

* **We jumped ship…**
* **We escaped via the underground railroad.**
* **We held slave revolts on plantations.**
* **We held a mutiny on the Amistad.**
* **We marched on Washington DC…(several times)**
* **We sat in at segregated restaurants.**
* **We passed "anti-discrimination" laws and sued.**
* **We rioted in the streets.**
* **We cried in the streets.**

BUT NONE BUT the CREATOR heard our cries !

> *Note: We will return to the Planet within one year to determine progress without us.*

==

The President of the USA fell to his knees on a pile of the newpapers and began shouting—

"NO! NO! No!!!!"

The President of the USA broke down and cried. He could not believe what he was reading. Worse, he could not believe that something of such magnitude had fallen upon the great United States of America.

SUDDENLY in his state of despair…the president could hear the voice of Connie calling him.

"Mr. President—, she called in a stern voice,

"please wake up. You are having a bad dream !!!

George Dubyah looked up and stared right into the face of his security advisor—*Connie*.

She said with a very kind voice,

"That must have been a really bad nightmare. You were yelling so loudly that you woke up a lot of people."

George Dubyah responded—*"Nightmare? You mean I was dreaming? There is no crisis of black people disappearing?"*

Then Dick chimed in—*"Well, yes the crisis is still going on—we are still trying to find out who is behind the* Anthrax *attacks.…"*

"Anthrax attacks!!??—what are you talking about !!?"

George Dubyah insisted to know.

Connie looked at Colonel Powell and Dick and then offered——

"I think he is still partially asleep. These recent terrorist attacks have probably caused George Dubyah. to be extremely tired and to have these nightmares. Let's get George Dubyah. some coffee and make sure he is awake before we try to fill him in on the recent developments with the Terrorists."

George Dubyah stared at them for a few moments and then came to his senses. He realized that this *MILLION FAMILY DISAPPEARANCE*—was nothing but a nightmare. He had been dreaming. He had awakened to the real events of Terrorist attacks that had been threatening the USA.

George Dubyah responded in a solemn voice.—"WOW!!!... *Do you mean it was all a bad dream !? It seemed so real. Are you telling me that we are not having a crisis of Black people disappearing ?*

Colonel Powell told him—"*Right now, sir, our night mare is a man named* Bin Laden , Saddam Hussein and other fanatics.*"

(Ignoring the comments about the Islamic fanatics)—

—George Dubyah told Dick, Colonel and Connie—

"*That NIGHTMARE WAS HORRIBLE—All the Black people had suddenly disappeared. It made me think——DO YOU REALIZE HOW MUCH WE WOULD NOT HAVE—IF WE DID NOT HAVE BLACK PEOPLE or many of the other people of color ?? I mean—think about it !*"

George Dubyah had been sweating during his dream, so he got up and walked toward the bathroom. He wanted to freshen up. But he continued talking about his nightmare——" *It made me realize how terrible racism really has been. It made me take a serious look at my own attitudes and actions. It made me see how important it is for everyone to be FREE.*"

Connie looked at Colonel Powell and Dick and then offered—"*God works in mysterious ways......Did you know that dreams come often come from the "spiritual realm of life?*"

She continued, " *Dreams can be subconscious reflections of what we really fear in life—often ignited by something that happens in real life. I bet that the threats to our freedom from the terrorists caused you to think about people of color who have had their freedom constantly blocked.*"

Colonel Powell asserted——"*As the great Dr. M. L. King said....a threat to freedom anywhere is a threat everywhere...*"

Then one of the African-American Presidential Aids spoke up and said:

"*Think about this—the first man to die in the Revolutionary War of 1776 was* Crispus Attucks—*(a black man)—and then the pilot of the* hi-jacked airliner that crashed over Pennsylvania a few weeks ago was also a Black man."

He continued talking—

Regarding this racial mess and the terrorists— good friend of mine told me something that really touched my heart. He is an older Black gentle-man who served in the U.S. Navy during World War II.

He said that he thinks that our country has been far too harsh in its treatment of the loyal, patriotic Black people.... who have fought and died in every War for the USA—but have been treated like second class pets—

And mistakenly —yet we have allowed foreigners—religious fanatics, criminals and every other type of trash—to come here (without question) and take advantage of our nation's wealth—and then turn on us and attack our freedoms.—while White America has been mis-treating the very people who built this great country."

Connie gave a nod of approval to Colonel and the Aide for their insightful comments and re-directed the conversation to the serious issues of the War—then asked—

"Do you recall that just yesterday before you went to sleep—that Osama Bin Laden had been shown on TV via a video and he was threatening a Holy War?"

Then the President asked, " *Yes, yes, yes—! What are the recent devel-opments with Osama Bin Laden—the evil one? I cannot believe he is call-ing this a* HOLY WAR*....when he treats his own people in Afghanistan so badly. I see nothing 'GODLY' about they way the* Taliban *treats its own citizens in Afghanistan."*

And Connie smiled because she knew he was now fully awake—and she responded, *"Well, Mr. President, he has threatened more attacks on the US –just like the ones of Sept. 11 on the World Trade Center. We have information also that he has not been acting alone in these Anthrax attacks. There are also reports that Osama is trying to buy nuclear weapons."*

"*Well, obviously, we have a major enemy to fight and they are not America's ex-slaves,*"——interjected the Presidential Aid.

Colonel Powell informed George Dubyah — "*So far we have some of the Taliban troops on the run over in Afghanistan…but we do not know if they are re-grouping or what.*"

The video showing Bin Laden's meeting where he was bragging about what occurred at the World Trade Center was about to be aired on TV. George Dubyah had to get ready for the news conference that was to follow the airing of this profound bit of evidence that Bin Laden was the culprit behind the attack on America.

After his insightful nap, George Dubyah was ready for another press conference, but this time, it was for real—in real life—concerning the terrible events of AMERICA'S NEW WAR against Terrorists.

The President opened his TV press conference with these words—

"UNITED WE STAND….*divided we will fall….*"

THE END

================

WHY SHOULD WE STUDY AND LEARN ABOUT PAST EVENTS? —
Author/historian John Henrik Clarke answers that question this way—

"History is a clock that people use to tell their time of day. It is a compass they use to find themselves on the map of human geography. It tells them where they are, and what they are."

COLLECTIBLE ARTICLE—#5

"GIRL TALK"

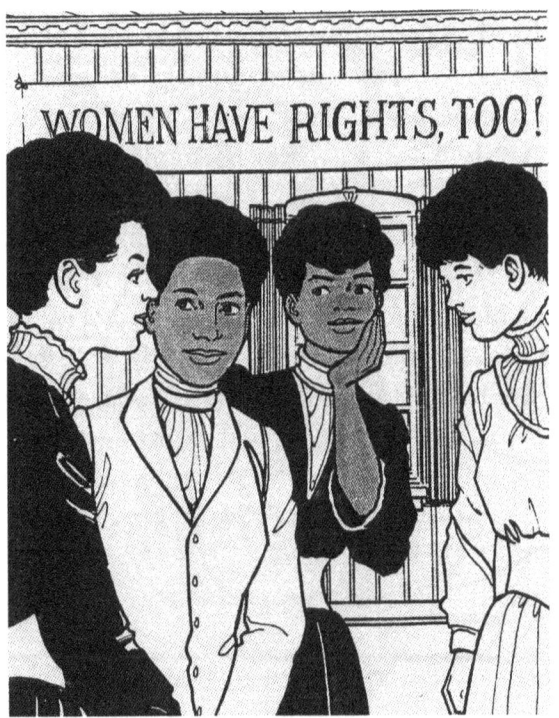

GIVE HONOR AND RESPECT TO WOMEN—
as they are your mothers, sisters, grandmothers, nurses, cooks, care-
takers and… teachers…."

The Godfather of Soul: James Brown made this popular song about women—

"It's a man's world—but it wouldn't be nothing without a woman or a girl…."

How right you are, Mr. James Brown!!!

All over this Planet, women have suffered at the hands of ignorance and cruelty, simply for being born female. It is one of the most barbaric conditions that exist upon the Planet.

Throughout history in the Middle East, Africa and the Orient—there are numerous incidents of injustices toward women. Why?

Perhaps because of mis-understanding of female ability and nature—or because of mis-guidance regarding what actually happened between Adam and Eve—women have been mis-treated throughout the world for many centuries. Eve was blamed for making Adam eat the wrong fruit in this old scriptural tale—and some folks actually believe that is the cause of man's down-fall. So women are blamed.

Because most Biblical and scriptural stories were written as parables or fables in symbolical language—it is certainly realistic to believe that this tale about Eve leading Adam to his downfall is not exactly true. But most people operate on some belief that women are "trouble."

Any arguments to the contrary are rejected—but it is highly possible that this traditional story of "Adam & Eve" is not accurate. Perhaps God is a GREAT SPIRIT. Perhaps God is a Black Woman. Perhaps none of this is true at all and there was no apple to eat…maybe it was all a symbolic story.

Women possess a power from birth that enables them to use the unique and amazing power of giving birth to new things and new people, creativity, flexibility, endurance, persistence, altruism, and love.

And the plight of modern women developed from a long history of mis-treatment of women, using females for sexual pleasure, and general injustice toward women.

The history of the oppression and mis-treatment of women is quite extensive. From the beginning of these United States, the laws and institutions were designed to create and maintain the privileges of WHITE MALES…principally rich white males.

While John Adams was involved in helping to write the Declaration of Independence, his wife Abigail Adams was not in full agreement with him. She wrote the following note to him in 1776—

> *"I cannot say that you are very generous to the ladies, for whilst your are proclaiming peace and good will to men, emancipating all nations—you insist upon retaining an absolute power over wives."*

And she was correct ! Women in the U.S. have had to fight for equal rights, for the right to vote, and for equal pay for equal work.

It seems that much of it is based upon false stereotypes—that women are inferior to men. The bad treatment of women was carried out because of men who wanted to have power over others. It was necessary for them to spread stories and propagate ideas of "female inferiority" in order to rationalize their greed for power.

FANATICS MIS-TREAT WOMEN

—Most of us have read the stories of the terrible treatment of women in Muslim societies, beatings, rapes, castration, and 2nd class citizenship. And many of these Islamic governments are nothing more than cruel dictatorships. Since the Taliban took power in 1996, women have had to wear burqua and have been beaten and stoned in public for not having the proper attire, even if this means simply not having the mesh covering in front of their eyes. They want women totally covered and unseen…due to some fanatical beliefs about FEMALE INFERIORITY. Even for those who are extremely religious…according to scriptures—Women are suppose to be the "help-mate" for men. Women are not suppose to be mis-treated, degraded, beaten or harmed in any way.

One woman was beaten to death by an angry mob of fundamentalists for accidentally exposing her arm(!) while she was driving. Another was stoned to death for trying to leave the country with a man that was not a relative. Women are not allowed to work or even go out in public without a male relative; professional women such as—professors, translators, doctors, lawyers, artists and writers have been forced from their jobs and restricted to their homes.

Homes in Afghanistan where a woman is present must have their windows painted so that she can never be seen by outsiders. They must wear silent shoes so that they are never heard. Under the Taliban regime, women live in fear of their lives for the slightest "*mis-behavior.*" Because they cannot work, those without male relatives or husbands are either starving to death or begging in the street,—even if they hold Ph.D.'s—

But let us not just focus upon the blatant acts of the Taliban and ignore the other vicious conditions that women live in each day in nearly every nation. In the USA…every 5 minutes a woman is beaten by her husband, lover, or father. Abuse of women and children is at epidemic proportions in some states. There are more "safe places to live" for animals—dogs and cats—in the USA than there are for women and children.

This same type of mis-treatment has been occurring in some underdeveloped African societies where women are forced to have their female organs mutilated.

And in older Christian societies, women were oppressed and many women where accused of being witches—and thus, burned at the stake because of men's fear of their natural clairvoyant abilities, their knowledge of herbs—and for other ridiculous reasons.

And we will never live in peace until we give justice and equality to WOMEN.

Just like an airplane needs 2 wings to fly properly, our society needs both males and females in equal roles in order to become a healthy, balanced society.

BECAUSE THIS PLANET NEEDS BOTH THE FEMALE AND THE MALE ENERGY TO FUNCTION PROPERLY, WE MUST GIVE WOMEN EQUALITY AND THEIR PROPER PLACE IN LEADER-SHIP......

LET'S HONOR WOMEN ALL OVER THE WORLD AND ALL THROUGHOUT HISTORY.

HERE ARE A FEW OF THE UNSUNG DYNAMIC FEMALE "SUPER SISTAHS"—

Dr. Leaky *(an archeologist & historian)* discovered the oldest known human bones of a Black African woman.—more than 5 million years old—which means she was probably one of the true mothers of creation.

SOJOURNER TRUTH was an ex-slave who helped other slaves escape from the cruel southern plantations via the Underground Railroad. She was also a fighter for the equal rights of women.

MARY McCLEOD BETHUNE—started a college with $5.00 for Black people, which is now known as *"Bethune-Cookman College"* in Florida.

SARAH BOONE invented the ironing board.

ROSA PARKS has become known as the *"Mother of the Civil Rights Movement"*—because she refused to give up her seat on a segregated bus—which lead to the famous Montgomery Bus Boycott.

MAGGIE WALKER—first woman banker in USA.

BILLIE HOLIDAY..."—blues singer....—was one of the originators of "Blues"

MADAME C.J. WALKER—self-made millionaire who created hair products & hot combs for Blacks.

"If it weren't for grease and a straightening comb—some of these sistahs would have to hide at home...."

(—an old popular verse regarding Madame Walker's inventions, chanted by many Black girls.)

Phyllis Wheatley became the first published Black American Poetess

WE APPRECIATE ALL OF OUR GREAT SUPER
SISTAHS WHO HAVE HELPED TO IMPROVE LIFE
ON THIS PLANET—

Marian Anderson
Susan B. Anthony
Lucille Ball
Mary McCleod Bethune
Gwendolyn Brooks
Shirley Chisholm
Sara Delaney
Flo Jo (Florence Joiner)
Betsy Ross
Florence Nightingale
Rosa Parks
Mary Church Terrell
Betty Shabazz

Mother Teresa
Sojourner Truth
Harriet Tubman
Sara Vaughn
Dina Washington

And thousands and millions of others fantastic women !!!
****

"HOOD-WINKED!"—

The Origin of Stereotypes"—

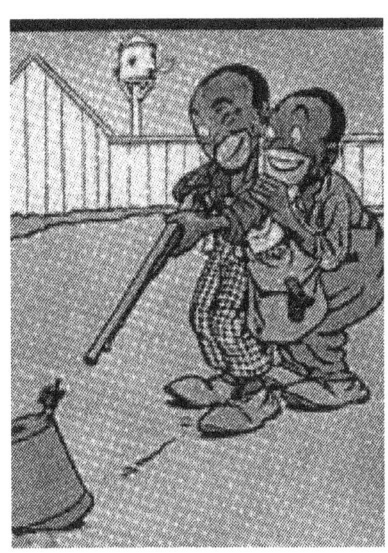

LITTLE BLACK SAMBO, MAMMY, COONS, PICKANINNIES, JIG-A-BOOS is what they were called——while grinning tap-dancers, Loyal Toms, carefree Sambos, faithful Mammies, grinning Coons, savage over-sexed black brutes, and wide-eyed nit-wits——rolled across the TV screen in cartoons, feature films, popular songs,—and appeared in books, minstrel shows, advertisements, folklore, household artifacts, even children's rhymes.

These ugly racial images and stereotypes had their origin in slavery—when White men had the need to degrade and demean Black people in order to rationalize their insane business of enslaving, segregating and abusing other human beings.

The "coon" caricature is one of the most insulting of all anti-Black caricatures. The name itself, an abbreviation of raccoon, is dehumanizing. As with Sambo, the coon was portrayed as a lazy, easily frightened, chronically idle, inarticulate buffoon.

The coon differed from the Sambo in subtle but important ways. Sambo was depicted as a perpetual child, not capable of living as an independent adult. The coon acted childish, but he was an adult—yet a " good-for-nothing" adult.

The coon, although he often worked as a servant, was not happy with his status. He was simply too lazy or too cynical to attempt to change his lowly position. Also, by the 1900s, Sambo was identified with older, docile Blacks who accepted Jim Crow laws and etiquette; whereas coons were increasingly identified with young, urban Blacks who disrespected Whites. Stated differently, the coon was a Sambo gone bad.

Sambo was portrayed as a loyal and contented servant. Indeed, Sambo was offered as a defense for slavery and segregation. How bad could these institutions have been, asked the racialists, if Blacks were contented, even happy, being servants?

African-Americans suffered for many years under the promotion of these degrading images of them…and many had to tolerate these forms of mental abuse just to survive and maintain an income.

Black actors who wanted to work in film were relegated to playing roles of 'stupid, lazy, unmotivated dummies"—who had bulging eyes, slurred speech and no ingenuity—such as the famous TV character:

"Stepin' Fetchit." and *"Amos & Andy."*

White people laughed at these images, produced products—such as toys, banks, dolls and other ugly souvenirs that portrayed these ridiculous, negative and degrading images of Black people. Some White people also participated in *"Minstrel Shows"*—in which they put black make-up their faces and made fun of African-Americans.

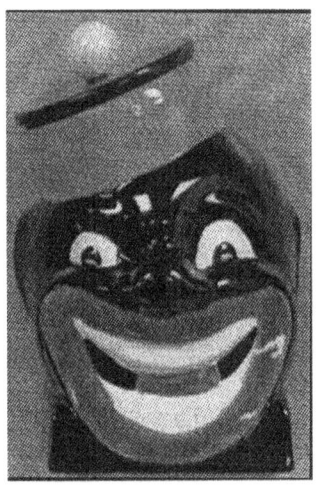

White people produced and sold souvenirs, banks, toys, and all sorts of gadgets based upon these degrading stereotypes of a "worthless, lazy, ignorant, unmotivated Black person."

White society ridiculed Black people as a group and in ways that were absolutely the worst degrading and dehumanizing to ever exist in the history of the world. All Black (Negroes) people were lumped into one group and ridiculed—across the board. It did not matter whether the Black person was actually an inventor, champion athlete, skilled musician or a teacher, a writer or a doctor. White society ridiculed the entire race of people. And many continue to do so into the 21st Century.

These dehumanizing caricatures permeated popular culture from the 1820s to the Civil Rights period and implanted themselves deep in the American psyche.

These degrading images of Black people represent some of the most painful experiences for Africans in the USA.

Likewise, many other people of color—minority groups—such as: Native American Indians, Chinese, Japanese, Mexicans and others have suffered under these same types of degrading mis-representations of them as a group of people.

Most people believe slavery no longer exists, but it is still very much alive. From Khartoum to Calcutta, from Brazil to Bangladesh, men, women, and children live and work as slaves or in slave-like conditions. According to the London-based Anti-Slavery International (ASI), the world's oldest human-rights organization, there are at least 27 million people in bondage. Indeed, there may be more slaves in the world than ever before. This fact is generally not known. In part, this is because modern-day slavery does not fit our familiar images of shackles, whips, and auctions.

Contemporary forms of human bondage include such practices as forced labor, servile marriage, debt bondage, child labor, and forced prostitution. Modern slaves can be concubines, camel jockeys, or cane cutters. They might weave carpets, build roads, or clear forests. Though the vast majority are no longer sold at public auction—today's slaves are often no better off than their more familiar predecessors. Indeed, in many cases, their lives are more brutal and hazardous.

MANY FACTS FROM HISTORY (especially African-American History)—HAVE BEEN "lost, stolen, and strayed..." AND OUR NATION CONTINUES TO BE EMBROILED IN DEBATES OVER 'discrimination'... 'racism'... 'affirmative action'...sexism, women's rights and reparations.

"When you make men slaves...you compel them to live with you in a state of war."

~ Quote from Olaudah Equiano Oil (1780)
—*son of an Ibo Tribal Elder who escaped from American slavery.*

LEARNING MORE ABOUT THE TRUE FACTS AND EVENTS OF HISTORY CAN HELP US TO BETTER UNDERSTAND WHERE WE CAME FROM AND WHERE WE MUST GO TO SOLVE OUR PROBLEMS.

THE TRUTH ABOUT BLACK HISTORY:

CONTRARY TO POPULAR ERRONEOUS BELIEFS—HIGH LEVELS OF WISDOM AND KNOWLEDGE ORIGINATED IN AFRICA.... SCIENCES, ARCHITECTURE, MEDICINE, MATHEMATICS, ASTRONOMY, HERBOLOGY, SPIRITUALITY—and many other wonderous fields, had their origins in Africa thousands of years ago—before White people ever went to the continent.

That's Right! As a result of cruel stereotypes against Black people and this false propaganda about "black inferiority"—many people of all races have been brain-washed to incorrectly believe that "race & color" are connected with intelligence or ability.

Africa was the cradle of civilization, where humans first created organized ways of living, schools, businesses, and the arts.

When the Greeks, Chinese, and Europeans first went to Africa, they found Black people who had high levels of advancement for the times. We must acknowledge that and learn from the wisdom of our ancestors.

The famous actor Dr. William Cosby (Bill Cosby) made a film that was titled: *"Black History: Lost, Stolen, Strayed"*—in which he pointed out the many instances where the true history of Africans Black people in general has been hidden, lost, distorted and confused by unjust writers and historians.

In fact, other groups of people, including the Native American Indians, Latinos, Orientals, and Aborigines—suffered from this form of racial propaganda. Many of those ancient writers from Europe did not understand the societies and cultures of the dark-skinned people that they encountered. There were many philosophical differences between the Caucasians and the other groups.

For example: The Native American (Indians) did not believe in "ownership of land by individuals." They had a totally spiritual view of the Earth. They did not believe in ownership of people by other people (slavery) either. The Europeans came to the Americas with the main purpose of capturing the land and owning it.

Even during the days of African slavery in the US, White masters would sleep with Black women during the night, would get them pregnant—and yet, kept them in slavery because of their insatiable greed to be in power. Many recent reports from historians have verified that Thomas Jefferson and other white American leaders did have children with black slave women.

The desire to enslave the darker people was the ultimate reason that racial stereotypes and lies were promoted. And unfortunately, many of these stereotypes still exist in the minds of modern people of the 21st Century.

SLAVE REBELLIONS:

The African slaves were far from being lazy, docile, nit-wits. There were many slaves who engineered escapes and revolts. The following is a brief list of some of the most noted slave rebellions.

1663—The first serious slave revolt in Virginia.
1739—Major slave revolt in New York—9 whites killed.

1741—Series of suspicious fires set in NY causing hysteria among whites…31 slaves executed.

1773—Slaves in Massachusetts petitioned the legislature for freedom. There were a total of 8 major PETITIONS during the Revolutionary War Period.

1791—Haitian Revolution began with revolt of slaves.

1811—The largest slave revolt in the US—New Orleans. Troops called in to suppress the revolt.

1822—Denmark Vessey organized one of the most elaborate slave revolts in history that involved thousands of black slaves.

REF: *Before the Mayflower*—by Lerone Bennett

CORRECT EDUCATION:

Dr. Carter G. Woodson spent many years studying and writing about the accomplishments, inventions, and achievements of Black people. He found so many (thousands) inventions & achievements and wrote many books about this topic. He believed that there should be a record of these achievements—because—if we do not record it—other groups will try to falsely claim the accomplishments.

He also believed that it was very important that Black people also learn about their own history and great heritage so that we can be properly educated and know the truth.

EVERY YEAR MANY OF US OBSERVE—*"Black History Month"* in February thanks to the efforts of Dr. Carter Woodson, who started this event back in the 1920's via getting a legal proclamation for *'Negro History Week."*

Our school textbooks and courses have also been partly responsible for perpetuation of some of the negative stereotypes—utilizing books, manuals and other materials which promote WHITE PEOPLE and ignore the contributions of Blacks, Indians, Women and other groups.

Most people can easily remember the lessons from elementary school book about Thomas Edison, Betsy Ross, Christopher Columbus, Robert Fulton, and many other Caucasian (European) achievers and leaders….and even Little Black Sambo. The typical school curriculum is filled with lessons about Europe and White people—but simultaneously—the achievements, events and leaders of people of color are seriously ignored.

Because of the poor level of education, biased history books, and white-washed media…many lies and false stereotypes have been perpetuated. Millions of people have been mis-led to believe that Black people are naturally (biologically) inferior—stupid, lazy, uneducable, and non-religious.

Ugly STEREOTYPES have been promoted against women, against Hispanics, Orientals and mostly against anyone who did not fit into the established *"White society."*

** *EXAMPLES:*

"The only good Indian is a dead Indian."
"A woman belongs in the kitchen—barefoot and pregnant."
"All Negroes are lazy and stupid."

RESULTS OF BIASED WRITINGS....

Many unjust historians have tried to distort the truth about Black people in Africa and written books that characterize Black people as "ignorant, wild savages."

And to make matters worse, many out-right lies were told in order to convince people of the propaganda that 'Negroes' are inferior to Caucasians (White people)…in order to rationalize the evil practice of an inhuman slave trade.

STEREOTYPES are lies and false portrayals of groups of people which have been used to subjugate and oppress various groups of people.

However, there are many other scholars, researchers, historians, and anthropologists who have studied this issue—such as: Dr. Louis Leakey, Dr. Walter Rodney, Cheikh Anta Diop, Joseph Ki Zerbo, and J.A. Rogers——and concluded that all life on Earth began with the Negro (black people).

SIGNIFICANT OUTRAGEOUS SCANDAL:

One of the biggest social scandals in the history of mankind is the issue of the chronic suffering and poverty of the African-American (Black) people and the destruction of Africa.

The descendents of these slaves have reaped very few benefits and have been subjected to other horrible treatment since *"The Emancipation Proclamation."*

Considering that the ancestors of Black people have contributed so many wonderful inventions, music, poetry, revolutionary machines, medicines, foods, and ideas to the growth of the USA and the world— how can it be justified that most Blacks live in a chronic state of poverty, suffer from lack of good education, live in the worst housing conditions available and do not have access to the best in health care?

From the beginning of the Slave Trade, white people from Europe and other groups have benefited from the free labour of black slaves, from the many inventions created by Black people, from the riches and commodities that were stolen from Africa—and in every possible way. White people in the US continue to benefit daily from the fact that this nation was literally built on the blood, sweat, tears and brains of the African (black) slaves.

The history of black inventors and achievers is a long saga of oppressed people overcoming horrible conditions to accomplish the "impossible."

RACISM IS A SOCIAL DISEASE:

Although most of us do not like to address this issue of racism, it is a mental and psychological disorder that has been haunting our society since before the days of the ugly, horrible Trans-Atlantic Slave Trade of the 1800's. It is a disease in the sense that it acts like any other disease, such as cancer or diabetes or arthritis.

However, this disease feeds from mis-information, negative stereo-types and lies. It involves a belief in "superiority" of one race over other races.

SYMPTOMS of Racism:

JUST AS WITH ANY DISEASE, THIS SOCIAL DISEASE HAS SYMPTOMS, PATTERNS, AND DETECTABLE TRAITS......

IGNORANCE....lack of knowledge, concern or awareness of other cultures, races, customs of ethnic groups, etc.—manifesting in Perpetuating, promoting, selling or in any way advancing the spread of racist memorabilia, racist ideas, or degrading propaganda about another race of people—either via TV, newspapers, books, training, teaching or tutoring.

Failure to read, study or investigate the issues.

DENIAL or cases of *"historical amnesia"*
..... nearly complete denial and avoidance of the facts that indicate that there are racial issues, disputes and hostility based upon racial beliefs. Refusing to talk about, acknowledge or accept the issues, facts and historical events surrounding racial topics. Cannot or will not recall any of the major events of racial hostility.

FEELINGS OF SUPERIORITY BASED UPON RACE....upholding ideas and concepts that one race is superior to another race simply because of the skin-color or other racial characteristics.

ECONOMIC HARM is generally perpetrated upon victims of racism.

RACIST BEHAVIORS AND ATTITUDES:

INTOLERANCE.....inability (or unwillingness) to tolerate other people of another culture or race....narrow-minded thoughts that there is only ONE WAY that life should be—and that way is your way or the way of your parents.

1) Refusal to accept ideas that are different from one's own ideas relative to culture, race, spirituality, history, etc.

2) ILLOGICAL THINKING…..lack of any reasonable or logical explanation for one's hatred, dislike or intolerance of people of other races and cultures different from one' own.

   EXAMPLE: "I do not like Chinese people because they have slanted eyes…."

3) BELIEF IN STEREOTYPES…..lumping people of a certain culture or racial group into one category and believing things such as:
   • The only good Indian is a dead Indian."
   • * Women belong in the kitchen, barefoot and pregnant."
   • *All White people are devils."
   • *White men are smarter than everyone else."
   • * All Black people are criminals."

Belief is such stereotypes can be reflected in one's actions and in the way that people treat others of differing ethnic or racial groups.

Usually modern-day racist attitudes do not come forth in a direct form—because of the Civil Rights Movement, protests, and other Laws that make out-right racial attacks difficult and socially unacceptable—people use other deviant behavior to express their racial hostilities in subtle, covert ways. Often times, these attitudes are reflected in actions that are just a detrimental or insulting as if one had used a verbal racial slur.

Any other types of SABOTAGE, ATTACKS, VIOLENCE or hostility—such as: *lynchings, gay-bashing, cross-burnings, etc.*—toward people of a racial or cultural group that is displayed simply because of intolerance for their characteristic, physical appearance or religious beliefs—is a form of RACISM.

One of the reasons that racism is very difficult to deal with, to get rid of or to alleviate is that most people are in a state of "denial" about this problem. Most folks do not want to hear about this problem, much less admit that we may be suffering from this social disease.

AN IMPORTANT INCORRECT IDEA THAT NEEDS ADDRESSING—
There now exists a common mistaken idea that says something to this effect—

"Negro people should be glad that the white people brought them over here to the USA."

NOTE:
….AS IF TO SAY….that WHITE FOLKS did the Black people a "favor" by kidnapping them from their homes in Africa, selling babies from the arms of their mothers, lynching them, beating them, robbing them, refusing to educate them, denying them the rights of being human, by promoting false and ugly stereotypes about the inferiority of Black people, or by forcing thousands of Black people to work without payment (no wages) to construct this United States of America.

THIS IS A VERY MIS-INFORMED, IGNORANT BELIEF. THIS ENTIRE IDEA IS BASED UPON THE RACIST CONCEPT THAT WHITE PEOPLE WERE SUPERIOR AND THAT BLACK PEOPLE HAVE MADE LITTLE OR NO VALUABLE CONTRIBUTIONS TO THE DEVELOPMENT OF CIVILIZATION.

IT IS A DEEPLY INSULTING COMMENT & CONCEPT TO BLACK PEOPLE WHO REALIZE THAT MOST OF THE MAJOR (SIGNIFICANT) INVENTIONS, RELIGIOUS CONCEPTS, MEDI-CINES, MUSIC, SCIENCES, ARCHITECTURE, ASTRONOMY, AND TECHNOLOGY WERE ORIGINATED BY BLACK (Negro) PEOPLE and their descendents... (either in the USA or in Africa).

THE AFRICAN SLAVE TRADE WAS NOTHING MORE THAN THE SYSTEMATIC ROBBERY, DESTRUCTION, DEGRADATION, AND OPPRESSION OF THE BLACK PEOPLE OF THE WORLD. THERE WAS NOTHING NICE OR KIND ABOUT THIS HORRIBLE ORDEAL.

And it is the White people who benefited from slavery—and it is they who should be happy and honored to have the Black descendents of the builders of this nation in their midst.

BELIEVE IT OR NOT—

THE HISTORY OF SO-CALLED 'NEGRO PEOPLE' (BLACKS) IS EXTENSIVE, DEEP, AND FILLED WITH INVENTORS, WRITERS, SCHOLARS, SCIENTISTS, DOCTORS, & ACHIEVERS—AND AT THE ROOT OF ALL HISTORY OF ALL CULTURES.

If the so-called "Negro" people had never existed, THE UNITED STATES OF AMERICA (as we now know it) WOULD NOT EXIST IN THE HIGHLY DEVELOPED STATE THAT IT IS NOW.... we also would not be able to enjoy the many inventions, artistic creations and the music created by this group. We would not have: such inventions as...indoor toilets and peanut butter—nor music such as JAZZ, ROCK & ROLL, BLUES, RAP, and many technological inventions.

The propaganda about *"Africa being a savage place..."* is simply not true...

In fact, human civilization began on the continent of Africa. The origin of medicines, architecture, biology, spirituality, herbalism, holistic concepts, astronomy, construction, plumbing, art, sports, sciences, mathematics, and much more—ALL BEGAN IN AFRICA WITH BLACK PEOPLE.

BLACK AMERICANS WERE KIDNAPPED FROM THE LAND CALLED AFRICA.... Packed tightly in the bottom of ships and brought across the Atlantic Ocean.

The following illustration represents how the slaves were packed into the bottom of these ships for weeks while they were transported to the Americas to work for free building up the "new world."

The KIDNAPPED AFRICAN people lived in filth, disease, and crowded conditions in the bottom of ships while the White masters enjoyed all the comforts available to them up on the top levels of the ships. Many of the slavers read the HOLY BIBLE while they transported the slaves in these ships.

One of the first slave ships was named: *JESUS.*

Graphic illustration of a slave ship:

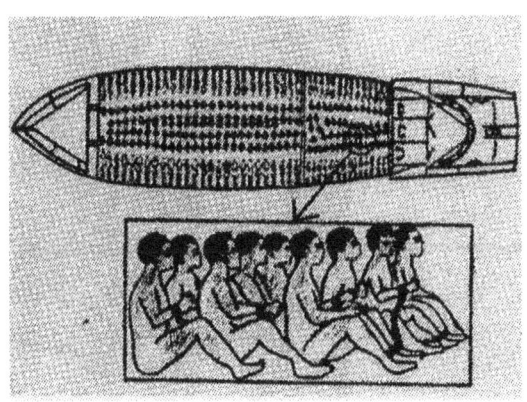

"..If the Atlantic Ocean were to dry up—it would reveal a scattered pathway of human bones—African bones, marking the various routes of the Middle passage."
~ Dr. John Henrik Clarke (author & historian)

DID YOU KNOW?—

In ancient Africa—Black people had their own civilizations, schools, temples, sciences, and many so-called modern conveniences hundreds of years before 1492 when Christopher Columbus sailed to the Americas.

And European explorers were not the first to find the Americas. Africans had been to the Americas and traded with the so-called Indians long before the Europeans thought of it. In fact, at one time in history, Africa was the *"New York"* of the world, where all new inventions, products, and concepts were found. Timbuktu was once the "mecca" for education.

Many run-away Black slaves lived with the Native American Indians. The so-called Indians were not racially prejudiced against the African-American slaves and gave them places to hide. Many Indians married Black people who had escaped from the cruel plantations.

Dr. Carter Woodson was up from slavery and went to college to become a PH.D. He wrote numerous books about the accomplishments and contributions of Black people to the civilization of the world. He is most famous for starting "Black History Month" observances in 1926.

VALUABLE Inventions & contributions

FROM BLACK PEOPLE

Garrett A. Morgan invented the first traffic signal and sold it to General Electric, which revolutionized the way we monitor our roads, streets and highways.

Invention/ achievement   *Contributor/ Inventors*

Air conditioner, incandescent light bulb;
Aeroplane propelling————————James Adams

And electric lamp————————Louis Latimer… (1886)

Automatic gear shift————————R. B. Spikes

Blimp————————J. F. Pickering

Blood & plasma preservation————Dr. Charles Drew..(1940)

Brakes & cable car————Andrew Hallidie

Clock (1st American)————Benjamin Banneker

Cell phone————Henry Sampson

Electric devices for railroads & trains——Granville T. Woods

Elevator————Alexander Miles

Hair softener & straightening——Madame C. J. Walker….(1905)

Heating & ventilation systems——David Crosthwait...(1925-1976)

Helicopter————————————Paul E. Williams

Ice Cream————————————Sambo Jackson

Ironing Board————————————Sarah Boone... (1892)

Mechanical & Air Brakes————Granville T. Woods

Pencil Sharpener————————John L. Love

Player Piano————————————J. Dickinson

Printing Press————————————W. A. Lavalette

Rotary Engine————————————Andrew Beard

Shoe stitching machine————Jan Matzeliger...(1883)

Toilet (indoor)————————————T. Elkins

Traffic signal & gas mask————Garrett Morgan

Typewriter————————————Burridge & Marshman

Dr. George Washington Carver invented over 300 useful products, medicines and treats from peanuts. He was also a famous "environmentalist."

AND WHAT WOULD AMERICA BE WITHOUT HER BLACK MUSIC? …*Jazz, *Blues, *Rock & Roll——and so on—the only true forms of music that were created here in the USA…. all originated in Black culture.
JAMES BROWN is the "god-father of Soul Music."
LITTLE RICHARD originated "Rock & Roll"…
ARETHA FRANKLIN is the "Queen of Soul Music.
HARRY BELAFONTE sold the first "million albums."

FIGHTING FOR EQUALITY:

The special examples of Frederick Douglas, Harriet Tubman, Martin Luther King, Jr. and Malcolm X *(& leaders of the Civil Rights Movement)* live on as part of this nation's rich cultural heritage for all Americans.
FREDERICK DOUGLASS was one of the greatest abolistionists who spoke out and wrote against the institution of slavery. He freed himself from slavery and began publishing an anti-slavery newspaper.

Thurgood Marshall won 29 of the 32 cases that he argued for "equality" before the Supreme Court.

BLACK PEOPLE HAVE FOUGHT AND DIED FOR THE USA:

The first man to die in the American Revolution of 1776 when the colonies were fighting against the British was a Black man——Crispus Attucks.

And there were Black soldiers in every war—from 1776 thru the Civil War and up til the present war on terrorism.

You probably heard that some of the passengers resisted the hi-jackers—but DID you know that the pilot of the plane that crashed in Pennsylvania (Sept. 11, 2001)——was a Black man (an African-American)........1st Captain Leroy Homer was a true hero! As a pilot,he refused to let his plane be used as a terrorist weapon! This act saved the U.S. Capitol,which was in full session!

Both the U.S. Senate and House of Representatives were in session! Not only did Captain Leroy Homer foil the assault on Capitol Hill, no one on Pennsylvania ground was injured! Now that is a heroic and outstanding act!…we also have an African American Hero= 1st Captain Leroy Homer

If it had not been for the Black soldiers who joined the Northern soldiers to fight—during the Civil War—we all might be using Confederate money today.

HARRIET TUBMAN is a woman that lead hundreds of slaves to freedom via the "Underground Railroad." She became known as " *A woman called Moses.*"

The TUSKEGEE AIRMEN were very instrumental in defeating the German Air Force during World War II.

Dr. Martin Luther King Jr. sacrificed his life in his non-violent battle for "equal rights" and for Americans to treat each other as human beings. His movement was the cause of many good changes in the USA.

All of these events—and more—have helped all Americans to enjoy more democracy, higher levels of justice, and the right to protest against injustices. Every year we celebrate and observe "Black History Month" and the birthday of Dr. Martin L. King, Jr.

======================================

NEWS REPORT:

MORE TAXPAYERS FALLING VICTIM TO
SLAVERY-REPARATIONS SCAM

OHIO—Nearly 80,000 Americans claimed a refund because of slavery on their federal tax returns last year, to the tune of $2.7 billion.
The only trouble is, the government has no such giveback.

Internal Revenue Service officials worry that a new wave of black Americans is falling prey to an old scam promising $40,000 to $80,000 in slavery-reparation tax credits or refunds.

Though scam artists prey mostly on the elderly and Southern blacks, charging $50, $100 or more for advice on claiming the refund, e-mail is spreading the word of the supposed refunds across the country.

Now there's new worry that promoters are going after other groups, too. About 200 claims have been submitted for American Indian reparations.

"This problem has never gone away," said Chris D. Kerns, a spokesman for the IRS in Cincinnati.

*(Article reported in the Afro-American Almanac News)

****

An old American Indian proverb says something to this effect…

"…do not judge another person until and unless you have walked a mile in his moccasins."

****

COLLECTIBLE ARTICLE—#7

"Holistic Healing"

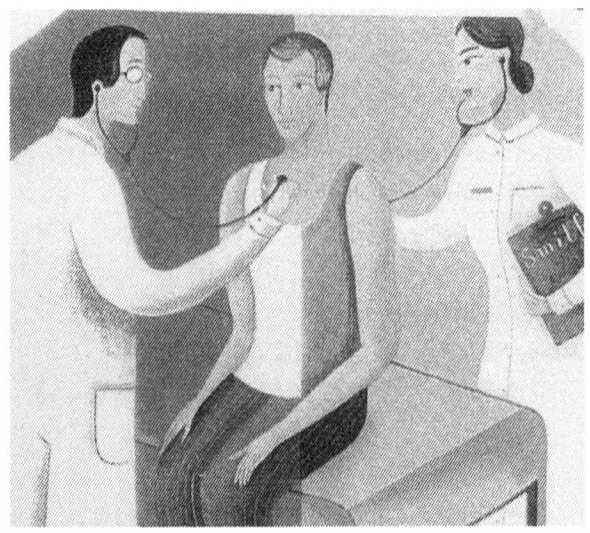

Moving toward healing our Planet....
—beginning with the person in the mirror !

This information is provided for your education and awareness. It is in no way intended to diagnose, treat or cure your disease. No magical cures are implied from this chapter. If you are suffering from an ailment, please visit a qualified health care provider, chiropractor, D.O. or other specialist.

Holistic (wholistic) healing is a concept that addresses body, mind, emotions and spirit—the whole person in the process of attaining a state of good health and happiness.

BALANCE IS THE KEY TO MAINTAINING GOOD HEALTH.

Throughout history, people have relied upon herbs, plants, oils and other natural (non-drug) plant remedies to treat their injuries, aches, pains, and illnesses. Native Americans (Indians)used herbs & plants for medicines. The ancient Africans also used plants and herbs to treat their ailments.

Herbs and plants have healing powers because of The fact that they contain concentrated amounts of Organic nutrients—such as minerals, enzymes and phyto-nutrients.

Our bodies will heal themselves,
—naturally—given the proper CARE, OXYGEN,
NUTRIENTS, SUNSHINE, WATER AND LOVE.

ANCIENT WISDOM ABOUT HEALTH & HERBS

For hundreds of thousands of years,—as far back as the times of ancient Egypt—people have been using herbs and plants to heal their ailments, to prevent sickness, to cleanse their bodies of toxins and to enhance their food. Archeologists have found residue of herbs on mummies.

The Native Americans (Indians) used special herbal teas to cure cancer. And the ancient Africans also used herbs to ward off diseases. Many modern medicines contain herbs.

Herbs are powerful botanicals containing special phyto-nutrients—that have survived the test of time and proven to possess powers to assist the healing process. Herbs simply offer the body what it needs to correct any imbalances and to rid itself of sickness. Given the proper nutrients and care—the body will heal itself.

USE OF HERBS:

WHEN USING HERBS, HEALTH PRODUCTS, & SUPPLEMENTS, IT IS BEST TO ALSO CHANGE YOUR REGULAR DIET TO INCLUDE NUTRITIONAL FOODS, especially fruits, vegetables and fish.

THE MORE FRESH, RAW (uncooked) FOOD YOU CAN CONSUME—THE BETTER. Raw foods contain essential enzymes that help the body utilize and digest all the other nutrients. Enzymes assist the IMMUNE SYSTEM also.

Take your supplements in moderation with your regular meals for best results.Change your bad habits—e.g. stop smoking,drinking liquor, eating too much junk, etc.

Some herbs have medicinal properties and should be taken as carefully as one would take any other medicines. Other herbs have miraculous nutritional properties, and must be used on a regular basis in moderation in order to build up the body's systems.

FOR YOUR ENLIGHTENMENT—

—BRIEF LIST OF HERBS (aka: Botanicals), NATURAL SUB-
*   STANCES, & PLANT REMEDIES*
*   (and their traditional/historical uses)—*

** ALFALFA= known as the "father of all foods"….
good for treating arthritis and joint problems;
helps blood disorders; bone disease; fights gangreen; good
against metabolic problems.

**ALGAE (blue green)= improves energy &
metabolism; stimulates & strengthens immune
system; fights depression; good brain food;
inhibits cancer, lupus, arthritis & dementia.

**ALOE VERA= helps heal skin rashes, burns
& wounds; anti-inflammatory aid; inhibits
infections and viruses; oxygenates cells; cleanses.

**BARBERRY= fights urinary tract infections.

**BLACK COHOSH= Estrogen (hormone) replacement
for women.

**BLOODROOT= fights gum diseases and dental prob-
lems.

**CAPSICUM (red pepper)= relieves shingles;
herpes lesions; & other skin irritations.

**CATNIP= calms nerves…a tranquilizer.

**CHAMOMILE= relieves stress; calms nerves; speeds healing processes.

**DANDELION= fights pneumonia & respiratory infections.

**DONG QUAI (aka: chinese angelica)= stimulates/heals woman's fertility and female reproductive organs.

**ECHINACEA= a natural antibiotic; fight colds & flu.

**ELDERBERRY= stimulates the immune system…inhibits colds, flu, & HIV virus.

**EUCALYPTUS= fights bronchitis; loosens phlegm.

**ESSIAC TEA= fights/inhibits/destroys cancer & tumors.

**FENUGREEK= aids sore throat & coughs; inhibits Diabetes.

**GARLIC= fights infections; decreases blood pressure; reduces cholesterol level; strengthens immunity.

**GINGER= calms swelling & inflammation.

**GINGKO BILOBA= improves oxygen flow to brain; helps memory and mental functions.

**GINSENG= promotes energy & sexual activity.

**GOLDENSEAL= inhibits infections, colds, flu.

**GREEN TEA= promotes weight loss; lowers cholesterol.

**GURMAR= stimulates the pancreas—inhibits Diabetes.

**HAWTHORNE= reduces risk of heart disease & stroke.

**ICELAND MOSS= inhibits HIV virus (stops AIDS).

**KELP= stimulates thyroid (helps weight control).

**KAVA KAVA= relaxes muscles; relieves tension.

**PAPAYA= aids and improves digestion.

**PEPPERMINT= relieves indigestion.

**SAGE= lowers blood sugar.

** SOMA= an herb that cures all diseases; helps with weight loss, and much more.

**SOY = prevents many sicknesses; strengthens immunity; helps fight/inhibit cancer. Good source of MSM.

**WITCH HAZEL= soothing for burns, scrapes & bruises.

**WHITE WILLOW= natural aspirin—(pain killer).

BUILDING A GOOD STATE OF WELLNESS IS A PROCESS....

LET FOOD BE YOUR MEDICINE...AND MEDICINE BE YOUR FOOD.....

MODERN SCIENCE HAS DISCOVERED THAT THE FOLLOWING FOODS HELP IMPROVE HEALTH....

**APPLES= inhibit tooth decay; detoxify; improve metabolism; helps pancreas.

**BANANAS= lower high blood pressure; good for soar muscles.

**BERRIES= help pancreas & insulin production; (espec. Huckleberry & Cedar berries).

**BROCCOLI= inhibits tumors/cancer; blood cleanser.

**CABBAGE= inhibits craving for liquor/alcohol.

**CARROTS= helps eyes; inhibits cancer cells.

**FISH= lowers cholesterol; relieves headaches.

**GRAPES= fight bacteria, viruses & tumors.

**HONEY= heals & soothes; attacks bacteria & disease.

**SPINACH=inhibits anemia; increases energy.

Why do these foods help improve health?
Basically, they contain essential nutrients, and they are filled
with ENZYMES & PHYTONUTRIENTS, which are essential
for healthy body functioning.

Foods contain basic "organic" minerals & vitamins. "Organic"
refers to nutrients that are derived from living sources—
as contrasted with "inorganic" substances (non-living).

Organic Minerals are essential to the proper utilization
of Vitamins. Vitamins operate in a synergistic manner
*(together).

"HEALING OUR PLANET BY CREATING BETTER RELATIONSHIPS"

In all that we do—relationships are involved. Relationships are necessary for us to live in society, to hold a job, to be a parent, to participate
in church or sports, and/or to conduct business.
    Regardless of your line of work, your situation in life, your race, sex,
color, or religion—you have relationships in your life.
The problem is the most of us are not very skilled in how to maintain
good relationships. This aspect has to do with how well we treat other
people.

In several research studies, including one conducted by the Carnegie Institute and another by the Bureau of Vocational Guidance—they found that most people (more than 80%) lost their jobs because *of inability to "get along with others."* They also estimate that at least 66% of business failures are because of poor human relations.

REMEMBER:

"Sticks and stones can break our bones,
and words can break our hearts."

———

—*WORST BEHAVIORS FOR GETTING ALONG WITH OTHERS…..*

* Manipulating and controlling with fear.
* Being bossy and domineering.
* Degrading others with 'put-downs' or snide remarks…harsh criticism.
* Threatening and harassing.
* Ridiculing.
* Begging.
* 'Kow-towing'…brown-nosing (& similar).
* Being a door-mat for others to 'walk on.'
* Sapping others of their energy & time…
…..to merely get attention for yourself.

In order to begin to escape from these destructive behaviors, we must learn to like ourselves. We must satisfy our own "ego-hunger" before we can begin to think about others. If there is friction and trouble in a relationship—there is low-self-esteem and big egos.

IMPORTANCE OF HIGH SELF-ESTEEM....

In good, healthy relationships—relationships bring a great deal of personal satisfaction and all parties are able to keep their own egos and self-esteem intact.

SELF-ESTEEM:

When self-esteem is at a high level, people are easy to get along with. They are cheerful, generous, tolerant, and open to new ideas. No one is trying to dominate the relationship or put other people down. Their need for "ego-satisfaction" has been fed.

They can even laugh at their faults, mistakes, and blunders. Their personalities are so strong and secure that they are willing to take a few risks. They take most obstacles in stride and persevere. They are able to think about the needs of others and offer assistance.

One of the biggest causes of disputes and broken friendships is NEGATIVE FAULT-FINDING CRITICISM.

Some people just cannot seem to refrain from making a snide, sarcastic or degrading remark to those closest to them. If you are looking for "perfection"—you can find it in the dictionary.

MAKE MORE MONEY...HAVE MORE FRIENDS... LIVE A HAPPIER LIFE—

The entrepreneur, teacher, business manager or politician who can master the art of good human relationships will multiply his finances & material blessings, and enhance the lives of others simultaneously.

Many companies that are making a lot of money—have become successful because they have learned to create good relationships with customers, clients, and employees.

Human relationships are critically important and the sooner we learn to "get along better"—the sooner our planet will become more peaceful.

IMPORTANT INGREDIENTS FOR GOOD RELATIONSHIPS ARE:

a) Open communication.
b) Honesty and integrity.
c) Trust and respect.
d) Ability to forgive and ignore small faults.
e) Willingness to help other people.
f) An attitude of gratitude.
g) High self-esteem
h) Mutual good-will.
i) A sense of mutual/equal partnership.

WHY DO PEOPLE FIGHT AND ARGUE?

Most of the time is it deeply rooted in the fact that one of the above-mentioned ingredients is missing.

THE CAUSE OF TURMOIL, CONFLICTS, AND PROBLEMS—

Many scholars, psychologists and authors advocate that the root cause of most of our social problems and bad relationships is our mentality (or level of consciousness)—patterns of thinking & acting. There are higher levels of mentality, which involve love, achievement, harmony, and success.

Basically, the lower levels of mentality are often called 'primitive' or 'animalistic'—and are the cause of most human turmoil. There are 3 levels of consciousness (ways of thinking) that result in most of our problems, such as violence, abuse, addictions, racism, hostility, war, etc.

The 3 Levels of Consciousness (behaviors) which result in human turmoil can be categorized as follows…

> a) Greedy materialism
> b) Sensation-seeking
> c) Power-seeking in order to dominate others.
> Desiring to control other people.

NEARLY EVERY SOCIAL, MENTAL, & HEALTH PROBLEM CAN BE CATEGORIZED WITHIN ONE OF THESE "CAUSES OF TURMOIL—

.…*FOR EXAMPLE—*

* Wife beatings are the result of *"seeking to dominate others."* (Power and control)

* Addictions are caused by *"sensation-seeking"* behavior.

* Racism is an act of both *'greedy materialism' and 'power-seeking.'*

* Over-eating (obesity) is rooted in *"sensation-seeking"* actions.

<u>WAYS TO IMPROVE RELATIONSHIPS—</u>

* Make other people feel important.
* Express appreciation & praise for small acts.
* Accept and Approve something in everyone you meet.
* Listen to others' ideas & opinions.
* Smile…don't be a chronic grouch.
* Watch out for hurtful words.

The entire issue of human struggles goes far beyond the physical world that we see and experience every day. We must remember that life is a spiritual experience—as well as a physical one.

****REFLECTIONS ON CARE OF THE SOUL…**

Soul is the eternal, true identity & essence—the true Self & sacred part of each person. In order to connect with the deepest and most real Self—we must allow our 'inner child' to become an integral part of our life.

Your eternal self—that spiritual aspect—your 'inner child' is that *'wonder woman'* or *'super man'* that lives in you. It is that creative self that causes you to regenerate and heal. Your 'inner child' is the truest reflection of the authentic YOU….*YOUR SOUL.*

We are not just physical beings seeking a spiritual experience—NO.

Actually we are spiritual beings in a physical body having and Earthly experience. Every soul is on a journey of liberation & God realization. Scholars believe that the Soul consists of several dimensions. The ULTI-MATE DESTINY of the Soul is to achieve full synthesis of all its components, which results in *"the Christ consciousness"*—which is actually the mind-set of Jesus when he had grown to a very high level of spiritual-ity—in human form. The stories told about Christ always begin with his birth as a 'golden child' who was ostracized by the world. This story is symbolically true of all of our 'inner selves.'

Buried intense emotions are often the cause of *"mental illnesses"*—for which psychiatrists give medications. However, drugs will not cure any of these problems. A cure will come when we learn to cope with our strong emotions, as these are issues of the heart.

The heart is very important because it is also the seat of the Soul. One can only rise to the highest levels of spirituality and health by cleansing the heart of that which causes disease—including the negative attitudes, bad habits, hatred, greed, racism, and poor nutrition.

The ancient people of Egypt (aka: Kemet) used the "ankh"——as a symbol of the eternal, infinite soul. They believed in eternal life of the soul. All of their art, symbols, and architecture reflected their knowl-edge of Spirituality.

Just as nutritional deficiencies/ poor diets & lack of exercise can con-tribute to or cause diseases——strong emotions, such as: fear, anger, hatred, worry, loneliness…(etc.) can also cause physical sickness—if they become overwhelming and out of control.

Emotions are one of the dimensions of the Soul. We cannot hope to maintain good emotional health if we lose the goodwill of relationships with others.

When we begin to examine our past history as a child and as a mem-ber of a certain group, we can begin to understand how we developed certain patterns of behavior and certain feelings. These patterns may or may not be beneficial for us as we become adults.

Many people are aware now that using good nutrition, herbs, vitamins, minerals, and natural remedies are best to help build up the body's natural immune system and to help the body to heal whatever ails it.

We must also remember that nutrition is an aspect of health that works in synergy with other healthy activities, such as exercise and positive thinking. It is not sufficient to just take lots of vitamins—without learning about the many other aspects of creating a healthy lifestyle.

The ultimate serenity & physical health can only be reached via a spiritual path & belief in a *Higher Power.*

Balance is the Key—

SPIRITUALITY AND HEALTH:

Many illnesses originated in our "spiritual life" because of our failure to be in tune with the universal order of nature and life. Ailments begin in the heart, mind and soul—and then manifest in other areas of our life, such as the physical and emotional.

Sicknesses such as *addictions* and *delusions*—begin on a spiritual level and then progress into other symptomatic expressions.

The *Bible* and the *Holy Quran* are medicine books for spiritual sicknesses. Nearly every scripture that was ever written by a prophet or guru is merely a prescription for living a healthier life and taking care of one's "soul." By studying, reading, and praying and learning how to live a better life—we can overcome illness that exists on a spiritual level.

There is an intimate connection between the BODY, MIND, EMO-TIONS, and SOUL (Spirit). That is why true healing must occur on all levels—in a Wholistic (holistic) fashion.

"You are not just your body! You are seven bodies of energy…"

~Quoted from Anna Harlas

(author of *SPIRITUAL ETERNAL ENERGY*)

HOW TO GET A NATURAL HIGH—

Take a few minutes and read these. Think about them one at a time
> >BEFORE going on to the next one………
IT DOES MAKE YOU FEEL GOOD
WITHOUT LIQUOR OR DRUGS.

1. Pillow fights with friends.
2. Laughing so hard your face hurts.
3. A hot shower.
4. No lines at the Super Wal-Mart.
5. Your first kiss with someone special.
6. Getting mail.
7. Taking a drive on a pretty road.
8. Hearing your favorite song on the radio.
9. Lying in bed listening to the rain outside.
10. Hot towels out of the dryer.

11. Finding the sweater you want is on sale for half price.

12. Chocolate milkshake. (or vanilla!)

13. A long distance phone call.

14. A bubble bath.

15. Giggling.

16. Listening to original "Motown sounds" from a radio on a hot summer night.

17. Slow dancing with someone you really like.

18. Eating your grandmother's cooking.

19. Playing cards (or board games) with good friends.

20. Going to the carnival with friends.

=======================================

"OUTRAGEOUS TERRORISM"

To fight over religion is very hypocritical—as one of the most basic principles of all religions is *"thou shalt not kill."* Killing one's fellow human being is wrong under every Holy Book,—all dogma, rules and principles of all religion.

These fanatics have referred to all Americans as "infidels" (meaning dis-believers)—even though there are millions of Muslims who live in the USA. Many Muslims were killed in this attack upon the World Trade Center too.

These barbaric Islamic nit-wits advocate that anyone and everyone that does not believe in the same religion or in the same dogma that they do—that they should be killed. Basically they have interpreted the meaning of "Jihad" to mean that they will become self-appointed assassins of anyone who does not follow their way of thinking or believing.

THE *HOLY QUR'AN* states that:
"To kill an innocent human being is as if killing the entire of mankind....and to save the life of a human being is like saving all of mankind..."

THE EXTREME CRUELTY of TALIBAN OPPRESSION OVER-
SHADOWS ALL OTHER CIVIL RIGHTS PROBLEMS IN THE
WORLD....

*Many people have been making an argument that this horrible terror-
ism has come upon our shores because "America deserves it." They bring up
every social problem that has ever existed in this country to try to rationalize the barbaric acts of the Islamic Taliban dictators.*

However, neither *the Bible or the Holy* Quran (or any other religious
books) condone this type of murder of innocent people

The Taliban has a bad track record of its own.

Yes, America has had its share of problems—racism, discrimination,
lynchings, racial segregation, and such. We must acknowledge that the
White folks in America (USA) have not been so nice to Black folks!!!
NO THEY HAVE NOT!!!! ...

But... let's hope that in the midst of these terrorist attacks we can learn
the true meaning of our U.S. CONSTITUTION and begin to live with
each other in more harmony and unity under a FREE & DEMOCRA-
TIC form of government, which is based upon the principle of—"all
folks were created equal.

It appears that when a tragedy hits our shores, we can come together
and unite—no matter what color, race, or heritage. But in other times,
we have difficulty living up to our U.S. Constitution that calls for
"equality for all."

Although some of the people of the Middle East may have many 'justified' reasons for feeling this way, or for hating the USA government—
these types of terrorist attacks will only promote more hostility and

violence. It is very unfair to characterize the United States as a "totally evil land."

The USA may have its problems, but it has been a leader in helping many countries, and in aiding people in time of disasters. The USA has been the place that many new technological inventions, medicines, and machinery have come into being that assisted the world in becoming more efficient and more humane.

The Immigration Service is over-loaded with applications for "green cards" and "visas" from foreigners who want to live in the land of democracy and freedom. Above all—the USA is the home of democracy and voting. We do not live under cruel dictatorships.

RELIGIOUS FANATICS are the cause of most of the debates and problems that exist in the world today. These fanatics earnestly believe that ONLY THEIR religion is the correct way of life. They have absolutely no tolerance for any other ways of thinking or believing.

And let us not forget that there are fanatics in all types of *'religious labels'*—including Christian fanatics and Jewish zealots—who have lost their sense of what is decent.

In past history, many wars were also fought in the name of Christianity, in the name of Judaism…and because of other religious differences.

And they must take a look at the corruption and abuse that exists inside their own societies. The Islamic world has a history of abusing girls and treating women like property!

So—it is very hypocritical for these fanatics to attempt to "pass judgement" upon the USA—when they themselves have serious social problems in their countries.

There is nothing written in the teachings of Jesus or Muhammad or any other Holy Prophet, gurus or any decent people's religion that directs people to kill each other.

Although many radical Muslims claim that they are acting in the name of God…their own holy book says something different—

Others have claimed that this war is based upon the exploitation of the Oil Industry and has very little to do with religion. This may be a more accurate assessment of the cause of these terrorist acts…money and greed. For many years the US and countries in the Middle East have had hostilities concerning the oil business.

When the US walked out of the recent *"Racism Conference"* in South Africa with Israel and refused to discuss the racial problems that exist—that did not help US relations with many minorities or with the Palestinians. But even this event does not warrant the killing of innocent people.

Maybe this crisis will open everyone's eyes as to how terrible it is to be terrorized and made the victim of violence—whether the violence is perpetrated by Islamic fanatics or by the Ku Klux Klan.

IF AMERICANS CAN BECOME UNITED (on the racial front) TO FIGHT AGAINST TERRORISM FROM OVER-SEAS, PERHAPS WE CAN BECOME UNITED IN OUR JOBS, SCHOOLS, BUSINESSES AND IN ALL ASPECTS OF OUR LIVES.

WAR—What is it good for???

Absolutely NOTHING !

"DO UNTO OTHERS AS YOU
WOULD HAVE
THEM DO UNTO YOU…."
~Quote..*This is the LAW of ALL the Holy Prophets !*

COLLECTIBLE WISDOM—#9

"Well Kept Secrets"

Most of us have been taught a limited amount of history of concerning how human life came to exist, and we were led to believe that human beings evolved from monkeys, cavemen, or savages from the jungles—into the modern, sophisticated people that we see today.

And some of us have been mis-led to believe that most modern inventions, mathematics, art, and civilization originated in Europe with so-called White people.

History, science and archeology do not support these concepts….and the facts show that this popular (narrow-minded) idea of how life began on Earth—is not the case!

Many scholars, scientists, and researchers believe that life began on Earth millions of years ago—and that humans did not evolve from apes.In fact, an astounding amount of research indicates that Human life began in other galaxies.

We have been trained to think in certain ways and to depend upon jobs, religious dogma, and psychiatrists.

And many of us have been taught that medical science is the only answer to our sickness. We are constantly bombarded with books, advertisements, and info that tell us that prescription drugs are the answer to all of our ills….while simultaneously—our society remains diseased.

Ancient societies did possess some secrets to long life, to happiness, to eternal life and to many of life's dilemmas. It behooves those who seek the truth to be open-minded and investigate these well-kept old secrets.

HERE ARE SOME OF THE WELL KEPT SECRETS:
SECRETS OF THE UNIVERSE

"Whatever Heaven ordains is best…"

~Quote from Confuscius

INFLUENCES OF PAST EXPERIENCES…

Within each person lies a vast store-house of experiences and feelings—failures and successes.

Those experiences are stored on the neural engrams (subconscious) of your grey matter (mind). Each one is as true as the other. The choice is yours as to which tape you choose to play back.

The past influences the present and the present does influence the past. We are not doomed to the past. These neural engrams can be changed or modified, much like a tape recording—or replaced.

Some psychologists would have us believe that past traumas, injuries and upsets are 'permanent damage,' but science has proven that this is not true. Old recordings, old patterns of thought, old reactions, old memories can be changed.

Because someone had an unhappy childhood does not necessarily doom him/her to be unhappy forever!

Our present thinking (mind set)—present mental habits, and our present attitudes towards those past experiences do influence and change what happens in the present and the future.

Discover your inner child...and you will also find old behaviors and feelings that are still effecting your life now. One of the best authors who writes on this subject is John Bradshaw.

DISCOVER YOUR INNER SELF:

BEGIN your own analysis by examining your childhood experiences....
*   Were your parents kind, supportive and loving?
*   Did you have a father who beat on you?
*   Were you forced to behave a certain way toward different races?
*   What did you learn to do to get along with others?
*   Did you grow up with an abusive parent?
*   Did you grow up with a parent who spoiled and smothered you?
*   What type of environment did you grow up in?
*   Were you taught to handle responsibility...or were you simply given everything?
*   Did you get your way by throwing fits when you wanted something?
*   Did you feel safe in your home?
*   Were you wild and uncontrollable in your youth?
*   Did you have to live in a racially hostile situation?

ANSWERS to these types of questions
will help you assess why you act the way
you do now as a grown-up person. It
will also aid you in understanding the
behavior of others.

All of these old behaviors may not be in your best interest in the real
adult world. Find out which ones are effecting you in your later years
that may be causing problems.

It is not about your age—it is about your attitude....how you react to
circumstances.

Your attitude helps determine your altitude!

By focusing our mind upon happy, positive, progressive, pleasant,
uplifting, healthy thoughts, ideas, concepts, and experiences—we auto-
matically diminish the effects of past traumas. If you choose, you can
put on a new
record and reactivate success patterns and feelings of joy.

UNIVERSAL LAWS...

Once we begin to understand the workings of the mind, the next step
toward living a successful life is to learn about
the universal laws... or *"Laws of Life."*

As we begin to understand these laws and apply them, anything we
want can be created. They are the same laws that govern Nature and
cause living things to manifest. The ultimate source of all Creation is
divine Spirit.

This Universe where we live operates based upon laws.

Here are 5 examples:

*"The Law of UNITY"—Everything in the universe is connected.
All came from ONE source.

*"The Law of GIVING & RECEIVING"—
We must be willing to give, in order to receive the abundance of the Universe in our lives.

*"The Law of CAUSE & EFFECT"——
For everything that happens (effect)—there was something that caused it.

*"The Law of RECIPROCITY"—
Treat Others As you wish to be Treated.
Some refer to this Law as *"The Golden Rule."*
This is another Universal Law that relates to the idea that you will get back that which you put out......The BIBLE states it this way—"*You will reap what you sow.*"

Some people explain this law this way: "What goes around, come around...."

*"The Law of DHARMA"—
which says that we all have a purpose.
The Ultimate Goal is to find one's Purpose in life and to blend that with service to others.

THE LAW OF LOVE—

ULTIMATELY—ALL OF THESE LAWS ARE BASED UPON THE SUPREME LAW OF LOVE. GOD IS LOVE.

The FUTURE BELONGS TO THOSE WHO
OBTAIN EDUCATION—
and WHO DO SOME SELF-ANALYSIS…

ASTROLOGY:

MANY PEOPLE BELIEVE THAT ASTROLOGY is a living science that actually effects and helps determine our behavior.

True science or not???—There may some level of truth in astrology because of the fact that energy comes from various planes of the universe. We are all "energy beings…"—and on that basis there may be support for the ideas that planetary energies effect us.

It is a fact that those who have studied "astrology" in depth have found many common patterns of behavior among people born on certain dates….

Most "experts" in this field of Astrology do NOT use it so much to try to predict one's FATE or the future or to direct one's life as if we have no choices,—but rather they use it to help analyze and assess one's entire personality, behavior patterns, and character. It has been well documented in books that some people born under certain Sun Signs do better in certain jobs or occupations than in others.

For instance—Capricorns are well-known to be enterprising, business-minded people. They are the "money-sign" of the Zodiac. Many Capricorns, such as Richard Nixon, and Muhammad Ali——became very wealthy and famous.

FOR EXAMPLE....

Each Sun Sign is classified into the following groups...

> AIR-=Mental
> WATER= Emotional
> EARTH= Practical
> FIRE= Ambitious

The following are some of the CHARACTERISTICS that people born under these Sun Signs have talents and personality traits exhibited in regards to.... for example= *"doing business"*—

*ARIES—Fire sign...aggressive; has new ideas; ...likes to become an authority or expert.

*TAURUS—Earth sign...likes a single focus & is hard-worker.

*GEMINI—Air sign.... Can do several things simultaneously.

*CANCER—Water sign..... Seeks security & stability in home-life.

* LEO—Fire sign..... Social worker-types; likes to help others; make good interpreters.

* VIRGO—Earth sign….. Meticulous, adaptable,—like cleanliness; enterprising.

* LIBRA—Air sign….. A negotiator for large groups

* SCORPIO—Water sign…. Intense; like to lead;
….. goal oriented & driven to success.

* SAGITTARIUS—Fire sign…. Analytical minded, tend to enter
the professions—such as Law or Psychology; generous & philosophical.

* CAPRICORN—Earth sign…. Very strong, intelligent; good organizers;… enterprising….loves to make money.

* AQUARIUS—Air sign…. Natural teachers/ trainers

* PISCES—Water sign…. Extremely sensitive; generous;
…. make good models, artists, decorators, etc.

==

Aliens:

Numerous legends tell tales of super-beings who came to the Earth, killed the Dinosaurs, built pyramids and created civilization.

*… Ancient Indians (Native Americans) believed
that extraterrestrials came from the skies and
taught them knowledge.

*...Nubians (ancient Egyptians) thought that
their kings & queens were offspring of alien
'gods' who came from other planets.

*...The Holy Bible cites several instances of
encounters with 'space ships'—
e.g.= *"Ezekiel's wheel in the sky."*

*...The Aztecs and Incas believed that
powerful 'gods' came from outer space and built
'landing pads' on Earth.

*...Some old religious scriptures speak of a
"mothership" that is circling the Earth.

* Scientists have discovered that the ancient
Pyramids of the Nubians and Egyptians (and others)—were
built in alignment with stars in Orion's Belt. The alignment is
so accurate that it could not be an accident or coincidence.

A modern computer was fed data about the measurements, composition, size, and location of the Great Pyramid in Egypt—and the computer calculated that it would take more than 100,000 slaves and 6 centuries to build such a structure based upon present knowledge and resources. Based upon these calculations, many people believe that the Egyptian Pyramids were not built by Earthly human beings, but rather these amazing monuments indicate the existence of master builders from another planet.

REF: *The Secret Forces of the Pyramids* by Warren Smith

Many scholars and scientists reject the popular *"Theory of Evolution"*—that claims that humans evolved from the apes. The religious concept of God creating man from dust is also challenged.

They based their rejection upon the idea that a super human race of beings migrated to the planet Earth millions of years ago—and did kill the Dinosaurs, created colonies of offspring (aliens born on Earth) and are responsible for the building of such mysterious places as " Stonehenge"—" Atlantis" and the Pyramids.

A Professor from a Soviet Science agency discovered the skeleton of a man who lived over 52 thousand years ago. Professor Otto Bader said that " there was nothing APE-LIKE about this skeleton—and in fact, there were indications that this man wore clothing that was similar to modern garments.

There are other mysterious indications of existence of life on other planets, of aliens coming to Earth—including:

- drawings in rocks of men in space suits.

- Statues of men in space suits

- The Blair Cuspid—discovered on the Moon.

- Huge stone monuments and heads of people found in places where it would seem impossible to transport such a large object.

- Pyramids that are similar in design in various locations in the world—such as Mexico, South America, Egypt, etc.

- The mysterious Great Wall of Peru and the amphitheatres carved into the ground in Peru.

Many other researchers also believe that there is considerable evidence that human life started because of space travelers who came from other planets and inhabited the Earth—millions of years ago.

REF: *Not of This World*—by Peter Kolosimo

Dr. L. S. B. Leakey discovered in Kenya (Africa)
fossilized human jaw fragments that were date as far back as 20 million BC.

REF: *The Observer;* "Man-like Fossils" (London Jan. 1967

Flight engineer G. Messiha discovered that a model airplane made of wood existed in Egypt over 2,000 years ago—predating anything done by the Wright Brothers.

Ref: *Blacks in Science*—1983

DO YOU KNOW WHAT ONE ELEMENT HAS DESTROYED MORE RELATIONSHIPS & created more DIVORCES, and CAUSED BUSINESSES TO FAIL, CAUSED FIGHTS, PROTESTS & BATTLES; RESULTED IN LAWSUITS; BROKEN HEARTS AND DESTROYED FRIENDSHIPS, and RESULTED IN LOSS of TEAM MEMBERS, and LOSS OF MEMBERS FROM ORGANIZATIONS ???

Have you ever wondered why attendance at your meetings have been dwindling down?—where are the members?—how come people do not come to my program or workshop???????

Have you wondered why the players on your team do not seem to perform well—or why they lack enthusiam about coming to practice?

Do you find that people have been avoiding talking with you and you cannot understand it?

Are you losing friends, clients and/or customers—but cannot understand why?

EXAMINE THE AMOUNT OF....

NEGATIVE CRITICISM !!! ☺...that is involved in your relationships—or coming out of your own mouth!!!

DO YOU REALIZE THE DAMAGE that your mouth can do to someone when it utters too much....."fault -finding criticism...?

There are some people who cannot pass a day without finding fault with their neighbors, boss, workers, congregation, students, relatives, co-workers, or with anyone who happens to venture near them. These *"fault-finders"* will nit-pick and find a way to say something degrading, foul, or negative about nearly anything. Some of these "fault-finders" are very skilled at couching their ugly remarks to make it appear to be something else. Even when disguised, the foul comments are just as hurtful.

There are parents who seldom give positive compliments to their children. They only point out "what is wrong with the child." And there are bosses who never praise any work done by their subordinates. Then these same bosses and parents cannot understand why people try to avoid them.

TYPICAL EXAMPLES:

Here is an example of a typical subtle verbal attack on a close associate= A woman just bought a new house and is taking her buddy on a tour....the buddy says:

"I like your new house, but you have a lot of dust on top of your refrigerator. You are nasty. Don't you ever clean?

Now, what was the purpose in giving this negative remark? Did it help anything? Did it make anyone feel better? Could it have been said in a better way?

HERE ARE MORE EXAMPLES:

A young teenager proudly announces to his dad that after much difficulty—

"Wow! I got my first "B" in Chemistry class.

So the sly Mr. Fault-finding father replies——

"Big deal!!!...it should have been an "A."

****

Coaches do it to their athletes....especially when a player does not know how to perform a particular action the way the coach thinks he should. Coaches are famous for their foul, degrading remarks—espec. after losing a game. Remarks from coaches are usually something like this:

"I am going to get rid of the whole damn lot of you sissies if you do not shape up and win me a game!!"

OR—"*Hey, Joe if you do not learn how to dunk this ball today— how about if we ship your lazy butt to Siberia? what is your problem—are you retarded???*"

****

AND—Teachers do it to students. *FOR EXAMPLE:* When a student is having trouble with a particular exercise—the teacher yells at the class—

"I am sick of dealing with you hard-head kids—you animals!!! This school is nothing but a zoo!!"

****

Mary tells a buddy that she is planning to start a home-based business. So—her buddy responds with a knife to the throat—

"Now just what makes you think you can do that? It won't work!!"

☻THIS TYPE OF SUBTLE KNIFING HAPPENS ALL THE TIME TO THOUSANDS OF PEOPLE.

Some of us were even taught to repeat this little verse—as a way to rationalize using negative criticism…..

"Sticks and stones can break my bones but words cannot harm me…"

THIS IS SIMPLY NOT TRUE>>>words can and do harm us.

Ever heard the phrase???—"Loose lips sink ships…"

Well that is very true. Too much negative, sarcastic, smart-alecky, fault-finding, gossipy, and/or mean-spirited talk—will destroy any relationship, kill an organization, ruin a project, cause hostility on jobs—and *sink ships.*

WORDS CAN DESTROY:

The knives of "negative criticism" and "fault-finding" that people try to stick in us each day are just as sharp and deadly as those made of steel—and used by assassins. Our society has somehow become conditioned that making mean, harsh, insensitive comments—is somehow good for us. Some people are very good at expressing direct negative remarks…and yet others do it in more subtle ways. Either way—the remarks do hurt the receiver.

Whenever someone says something that is intended to make the other person feel *less adequate, incompetent, stupid, lazy, bothersome, ugly, odd, racially inferior,degraded*—etc.—this can be like stabbing them with a knife. If done enough times— it can become very harmful to the entire relationship.

For far too long we have tried to rationalize the use of these *NEGATIVE REMARKS*—as being somehow necessary to get people to act a certain way—or *"to motivate others.…"*

But MANY OF US USE these negative comments and descriptions *(not just coaches, bosses, or teachers)*———in our daily interactions———only to cause resentment and hurt feelings. Think about it!! Does the person being criticized and degraded know how to do anything better or faster (or in any different manner) than s/he did before the fault-finder trounced him/her with negative criticism??? Do you get better results when you blast someone's self-esteem?

NEGATIVITY causes the receivers of these ugly comments to want to stay away from the one throwing the knives. Bosses and supervisors use these degrading remarks to "reprimand" their employees—and often end up with a less motivated worker than before they made the remarks.

Use of racial slurs are also harmful. Most of us know the ugly *"N-word"* has caused controversy and fights for hundreds of years. There is nothing nice, acceptable or healthy about referring to another human being in a degrading manner, using ugly racial slurs to describe them. We have all watched the inner city riots and protests that arose because of the use of demeaning racial slurs in this society. There are many of these ugly racial slurs...such as: *"chink"* for Orientals; *"wet-back"* for the Mexicans; and *"camel-jockey"* for Arabs——something foul and degrading for nearly every ethnic group.

When words are used to degrade, tear down, demean, or point out someone's flaws and faults—constantly—or in a sour or foul manner—it certainly does hurt!!

People who sit up and nit-pick and someone's little flaws—some imperfection, some speck of dirt, *(under the disguise of honesty)*—are actually being very cruel——and are actually doing no one any favors. Everyone has flaws. If we spend time trying to find all of them—we would waste many good hours.

NEGATIVE CRITICISM is in an over-abundance in this society....on TV, on radio and in the classrooms. Our buddies want to use negativity to tell us what is wrong with our lives. Our parents use negative comments in order to "keep us in line." Teachers and coaches often degrade us for not being perfect.

> PEOPLE LIKE TO DISH IT OUT——but most people do not like NEGATIVE CRITICISM and few can take it.
> And likewise that element that can cause building of relationships and *LOVE TO GROW, MEMBERSHIPS TO INCREASE*

IN ORGANIZATIONS, LONG-LASTING FRIENDSHIPS, MARRIAGES TO BE FULFILLING AND MOST FOLKS TO BE HAPPY is=

❀ POSITIVE VALIDATION—

IF YOU WANT TO BE HAPPY FOR THE REST OF YOUR LIFE, TO BE SUCCESSFUL IN YOUR RELATIONSHIPS, TO ATTRACT PEOPLE TO YOUR MEETINGS, TO HAVE FUN WITH YOUR FAMILY.....etc.

It is time to learn the ART OF POSITIVE VALIDATION and

HOW TO WIN FRIENDS AND INFLUENCE PEOPLE....

People respond in a good way to affection, acceptance, positive recognition, training, education, support, positive remarks, rewards, and incentives.

THINK ABOUT WHAT YOU ARE SAYING TO OTHERS— —is it really necessary? is it helpful? is it supportive?—or is it degrading?

The ancient Egyptians also were the first practitioners of Herbal Medicines and Holistic Healing methods.

Archeologists insist that based upon overwhelming evidence that Black Africans were the first people to inhabit the planet Earth and utilize utensils—Negroid people created, designed and used all types of mathematics, sciences, and arts—and did build homes, use plumbing, medicines, music, and other aspects of civilization.

REF: *Black Man of the Nile*—by Dr. Ben Jochanan

Karate, Judo, Kung Fu, Yoga and other forms of Martial Arts were first founded in Egypt and other parts of Africa. Old records of such kicking, throwing, disciplined physical prowess—have been found in places in Africa and represent the foundation for modern forms of Martial Arts.

REF: *African Roots in Martial Arts*—by Kilindi Iyi (1985)

All aspects of this Creation have significance on 3 levels:
PHYSICAL, MENTAL, & SPIRITUAL.

**For example—*

"AIR" also is symbolic of *'breath of life or the spirit.'*

"FIRE" represents truth, passion, & knowledge, education, & light.

"EARTH" is symbolic of the physical universe & flesh, 'Mother Nature,'… mountains, etc.

"WATER" is symbolic of morals, emotions, motion & cleansing power.

Africans (Negro people) were smelting iron and building boats—and had traveled around the world to the "Americas" long before any Europeans (such as Christopher Columbus) ever left their shores.

REF: *They Came Before Columbus*—by Ivan Van Sertima 1976

The secret of personal success is staying in touch with your inner self, inner peace, joy and confidence."

REF: John Gray (author)

"Life was never meant to be a struggle, just a gentle progression from one point to another—much like walking through a valley on a sunny day. Look at Mother Nature. It expends a certain effort in sustaining itself—but does not struggle. If you accept full responsibility for your life, you will accept that your destiny is created by you. By having the courage to identify and face the causes of struggle in your life—you grant yourself the power to transcend. Once you accept that YOU ARE THE CAUSE (your attitudes, actions, and behavior) of the difficulties——in time, you can eliminate the struggles."

REF: *Life Was Never Meant to be a Struggle*—
by Stuart Wilde

"Insufficient Oxyen (to the cells) means insufficient biological energy that can result in anything from mild fatigue to life-threatening diseases. The link between insufficient oxygen and disease has been now firmly established."

REF: Dr. W. Spencer Way—(Journal of American Assoc. of Physicians)

MENTAL ILLNESS CAUSED BY POOR NUTRITION....

Further, many problems that appear to be *"mental illnesses"* are actually rooted in nutritional deficiencies.

Many *"psychiatric difficulties"* or emotional ailments have been mistakenly diagnosed and treated as a clinical mental problem, when actually they are the direct result of nutritional deficiencies.

*EXAMPLES:

1—DEPRESSION…is more often than not caused by a lack of specific hormones, neurotransmitters, and nutrients to the brain.Remedies such as:
St. John's Wort, "B-vitamins"; Amino acids, Super Blue Green Algae, seritonin, and minerals have been proven to be helpful against Depression.

2—INSOMNIA…is often diagnosed as a 'psychiatric symptom' with other labels for diseases. Remedies such as…Kava Kava and 'Malic Acid' are good, natural relaxants.

3—DEMENTIA & MEMORY PROBLEMS…often the elderly are plagued by this problem, which can be helped with remedies such as: *"Gingko Biloba."* There are many natural (herbal) foods for the strengthening of the brain…including Super Blue Green Algae.

4—(ADD)—HYPERACTIVE CHILD—ATTENTION DEFICIT DISORDER…more often than not—children who have been diagnosed with this problem suffer from poor diets filled with junk foods. Remedies for this problem include…eating more raw fruits & vegetables, brain foods—such as Algae and Soy, and amino acids. Any natural remedy that enhances 'neuro-transmitters' in the brain will be helpful for this condition.

REMEMBER...

Each organ & all tissues of the body (heart, lungs, stomach,etc.) utilizes certain vitamins, minerals, proteins and
other nutrients in order to properly function. If your body
becomes deficient in certain nutrients, then these organs
lose their life force and some of the following problems
may manifest.....
refer to the following chart:

DEFICIENT ORGAN: RESULTING PROBLEMS:

*Liver————————————anger, hostility
*Stomach————————————gullibility
*Gallbladder————————resentments; grief
*Heart————————————Co-dependency
*Throat————————————debilitating beliefs
*Brain——————————Depression/Mood swings.

This is totally reasonable in view of the research that indicates that there is an intimate connection between the
BODY, MIND, EMOTIONS AND SPIRIT.

Good natural remedies for mental illness and emotional difficulties are
"Flower Remedies" and "aromatherapy."

And OXYGEN IS AN EXCELLENT REMEDY FOR ALL TYPES OF
SICKNESSES.

Low fat diets do not work. Most of the diet programs, products and plans that are on the market simply do not help the average person to lose weight. The truth about the problem of obesity and weight control is that SUGAR causes the production of insulin, which keeps one from losing weight. No matter how much one exercises, or eats vegetables, or restricts the intake of calories—the problem is SUGAR.....white table sugar.

If you cut the consumption of sucrose, weight loss will occur.

REF: *Sugar Busters*—by Dr. M. Bethea, Dr. L Balart, *et. al.*

FAMOUS QUOTES ABOUT HEALTH:

"Surely We created you of dust, then of a sperm drop, then of a blood clot, then of a lump of flesh—and then beholdest the Earth blackened— then when we send down water upon it—it quivers and swells and puts forth herbs of every joyous kind."
~Holy Qur'an 22:5

"And God said, Behold I have given you every herb bearing seed, which is upon the face of the Earth, and every tree in which is the fruit of a tree yielding seed—to you it shall be for meat. And to every fowl of the air and to every thing that creepeth upon the Earth, wherein there is life—I have given every green herb for meat; and it was so."
~Genesis 1:29-30

"The health of the people is really the foundation upon which all their happiness and all their powers depend."
~Benjamin Disraeli

"Look to your health; and if you have it—praise God—and value it next to a good conscience; for health is the 2nd blessing that we mortals are capable of; a blessing that money cannot buy."
~ Izaak Walton

"Better is a dinner of herbs where there is love—than a stalled ox and hatred therewith."
~Proverbs 15: 17

"When the head aches, all the body is out of tune…"
~Cervantes

"He causeth the grass to grow for the cattle and herb for service of man: that he may bring forth food out of the Earth."
~Psalms 104: 14

"The cell is immortal. It is merely fluid (water) that degenerates. Renew this fluid at intervals and give the cells what they require for nutrition—and as far as we know the pulsation of life may go on forever."
~Dr. Alexis Carrel (Nobel Prize Winner)

ANCIENT PREDICTIONS:

Nostradamus has achieved an amazing track record for the accuracy of his predictions.

The famous clairvoyant prophet NOSTRADAMUS made many predictions that have come true… including the fact that 2 winged-birds would crash into 2 tall buildings in America. Some believe that this was a prediction of the Sept. 11, 2001 incident at the World Trade Center.

Many religions believe that there will be a final war between good and evil and that a horrible "anti-Christ" will come into existence just before that time of the end. Nostradamus predicts that this anti-Christ will be around for 27 years.

Nostradamus has also predicted that there would be a major FINAL WAR (The War of Armageddon).

He said that there would be 7 signs of this time:

1. Decline in faith of the 3 major religions and an increase in beliefs in bizarre cults, atheism, and false gods.
2. Revolutions, internal upheaval and turmoil in Europe.
3. Wars and rumors, terrorism, and disputes and rumors of war all over the world.
4. Massive famines.
5. Pollution of the Earth
6. Devastating Earthquakes and serious bad weather conditions.
7. World-wide plagues and diseases

Nostradamus also predicts that Armageddon will occur near the time that Halley's Comets passes by the Earth again. This comet passes by our skies every 75 years and is due to return in 2061.

But following the doom, gloom, earthquakes and destruction, Nostradamus also had high visions of a new world that was spiritual— a new religious awakening that lies just around the corner.

Nostradamus wrote:

"The divine word will give to the sustance (that which) contains heaven and earth—occult gold in the mystic act. Body, soul and spirit are all powerful. Everything is beneath his feet, as at the seat of heaven." (CIII-Q2)

Nostradamus wrote extensively about a future time of spiritual awakening and religious growth.

REF: *Nostradamus*—by Bernie Ward…(Globe Digest)

FROM THE BOOK: *"Lights of Guidance"*—*Bahai Faith*

page 532:

"The Negro race has been, and still is, the victim of unjust prejudice, and it is obviously the duty of every Baha'i, Negro or White, to do all in their power to destroy the prejudices which exist on both sides. They can do this not only by exemplifying the true Baha'i spirit in all their associations and acts, but also by taking an active part in any progressive movements aimed at the betterment of the lot of those who are under-privileged, as long as these movements are absolutely non-political and non-subversive in every respect."

****

*"A great discovery of any generation is
that human beings can alter their lives by
altering the attitudes of their minds...."*

~ Albert Schweitzer

****

COLLECTIBLE STORY—#10

"THE HOUSE THAT SLAVERY BUILT"

This story begins in Middletown, Indiana—a city that has been proclaimed by scholars as "the typical American city." Several books have been published about Middletown, but none like this one.

This story is true—except that the names have been changed to protect the innocent.

INTRODUCTION

In 1924 and 1925 studies were conducted in the small industrial city that later became well-known as *"Middletown USA."* This was one of the first scholarly works to attempt to describe the culture and social environment of a typical American city. Helen and Robert Lynd published 2 books, based on these studies, titled: *"Middletown"* (1929) and *"Middletown in Transition"* (1937).

Those authors described Middletown as a *"good specimen of American culture..."* Middletown is a small city in eastern Indiana on the White River, 54 miles northeast of Indianapolis, IN. They described the Teacher's College as one that would grow into a major University.

Forty years later, another group of scholars went back to Middletown and repeated additional studies. They wrote a book titled: *Middletown Families* (1982).

These books discuss the following topics in scholarly ways:

- *Religion and the Family*
- *Working Women*
- *The class system*
- *Sex and Marriage*

However, little mention is given to the conditions or life-style of the African-American citizens who live in Middletown. The only major comment made in all of these studies states, *"There is a surplus of black children and a deficit of young black adults...."*

This factor was attributed to the lack of decent jobs available to Blacks in Middletown. Unfortunately these books do not examine the plight, history or conditions of Middletown's Black population. During the time that the Lynds conducted their studies, this city's government was operated by the Ku Klux Klan. Middletown was plagued by racial turmoil, protests, and segregation. The African-Americans who lived in Middletown often called it *"Dodge City"*—likening it to the famous cowboy TV show.

The stories in our book *Ship-Ahoy* are derived from the diary and memoirs of our super-hero ...Melina...who became known as: *"Super Sistah."* Because of her exceptional writings that she did about the situation. Since Melina was born and raised in Middletown, they are her actual accounts of events that took place in Middletown USA. The stories are true...but some of the names have been changed to protect the innocent.

EPISODES FROM THE BOOK:

SECTION 1—

"The Adventures of Super Sistah"

PICTURE IT——Middletown, Indiana 1948:

Our story begins in 1948 in Middletown, Indiana on a cold December evening when an African-American baby girl was born to *Mr. & Mrs. Melanin Milner.* They named their baby girl Melina. Melanin and Liza Milner were the descendants of run-away slaves out of Kentucky. Her great-grandparents had escaped from a plantation and lived with Indians.

This couple lived on the side of town called: *"Brownly"*
—where all Black people were forced to live. Most White people lived on one side of town and any other minority groups *(e.g.—Mexicans, Africans, Puerto Ricans, etc.)* were permitted to live only in certain sectors. Racial segregation was the rule of law in those days.

This town became known as *"Dodge City." (among blacks)*

Middletown was a wild city in those days....filled with gamblers, gangsters, prostitution, and worse!! Crime flourished in Middletown. Mobsters—such as *Dillinger*—were known to be active or heavily invested in Middletown's *'red light district.'*

For the most part—the Black folks in Middletown operated their own stores, barber shops, restaurants, cleaners, and other businesses. There were several African-American churches in Middletown...

The city government for Middletown was run by the Ku Klux Klan and the area was known to be strong-hold for racist activities, lynchings, shoot-outs, boot-leg liquor, and worse. Middletown held its Black population in virtual captivity and controlled the illegal funds as well as the legal jobs. White people were in power and the Black people had to find their own ways of surviving.

FAMILY LIFE:

Melina's family eventually grew....she had a baby sister named Karo, born 2 years after Melina's birth...Then her wonderful mother and father were blessed with a son, named Juan.

And later in life, along came the baby girl—Abby. Melina loved her family dearly—and helped to take care of the younger siblings. Since Melina was the oldest child in the family, she soon took on the role of "protector" for her other siblings. She was very helpful to her mother, taught her brother to walk and ride a bike, did errands, and generally helped around the house with chores. Her little sister Abby followed her around from the time she was 2 years old.

Grandpa and Grandma Milner lived only a few blocks away and they were farmers who were "share-cropping" on land owned by a White man, because the law did not permit Black people to own a farm in Indiana then. So, he farmed for another man, and was able to bring home plenty of fresh food for his own family.

Melina grew up on the poor black side of town. The houses there were basically little wooden boxes...nothing fancy. Middletown is in the midst of the 'cornbelt' and there were plenty of fields of vegetables...—such as *tomatoes, lettuce and corn*—growing all around Whitely.

Most of the Black people grew their own vegetables and ate the fruits from the trees. And many of them traded foods with each other. Food was often used as "money" between neighbors in order to trade for other objects that they wanted. Gardens, food and plants were a significant influence in her life from the time she was a very young girl. She enjoyed gardening in her own back yard.

One of the most popular forms of entertainment was to go fishing in *"Clear River."* Melina and her entire family often packed up a lunch, chairs and poles and spent most of the day on the river bank. The river was so clear that they could look straight into the water and see the bottom, see fish and other creatures which swam in the river. Upon their return home, their father would clean the fish and cook them for a delicious dinner. Fish was one of Melina's favorite foods.

Melanin Milner had served in the U.S. Navy during World War TWO…where he experienced terrible acts of racism from his own fellow sailors.

Mel returned home to his country only to meet with more discrimination. Middletown was like many southern towns in Mississippi, Nevada, or Florida—or other parts of the USA where racial segregation was the rule.

A FATHER'S EXPERIENCES:

On a hot summer night in 1990. Liza and Melanin Milner were sitting in their living room with a news reporter from the local Black newspaper: *"Middletown Negro Times."* The reporter was interviewing Mr. Milner for an article for *Black History Month.* Melanin was recalling tales of his experiences as a Black man in the United States Navy during World War II.

> *The reporter asked:*
> "Do you think that society has changed much since 40 years ago when you were in the Navy?

> *To which Melanin replied:*
> "Well, the white folks took down those insulting signs—you know the ones that said stuff like: *"NO COLORED ALLOWED HERE"* and *"WHITE ONLY."*

REPORTER: So you are saying that the social changes regarding segregation and racism have been superficial?

MEL: Yeah!!!—like I said—they took down the signs. We can now sit in the same bathroom on a toilet in a stall next to white folks. More black folks are in certain jobs....but the improvements are very limited. There is still a lot of racial hostility."

REPORTER: So—since you served in the military for this country...do you feel that it was well worth it?

MEL: NO! We black folks still do not have many freedoms like other people do. Just look at the way most blacks live in poverty and get discriminated against when trying to open a business or get a job. And black people fought for America in every single war since 1776. When I was in the Navy—the black men were separated from the white sailors. We were fighting for democracy and freedom that we have never had ourselves.

REPORTER: Tell me more about those experiences in the Navy—about the racial segregation....

MEL: Well, for example, one time the US Navy had loaded a bunch of us sailors onto a train to ride across the country to be shipped out. The white sailors sat in the comfortable part of the train and they put the black sailors in cargo. When it came time to eat—the white sailors were served real food and could get food from stores when we stopped. But the black sailors were only given left-overs. Many times we went hungry. The stores would not serve us either when we stopped.

REPORTER: Now that WWII has been over for more than 40 years—do you think it was worth it—would you do it again?

MEL: You must be smokin' something ! Heck no!!! I came back to America after all that mess overseas and I still have not had my full rights as a citizen. If Hitler's Mama was revived and started another war—I would not serve.

With that comment, everyone in the room laughed loudly. The room was filled with Liz and Mel's children: Melina, Karo, Juan, and Abby. There were also a few neighbors there to listen.

Melina was subjected to considerable amounts of racial hostility, she eventually developed even stronger powers of insight—and was able to detect injustice, racism and even the most covert forms of unfairness. She became increasingly convinced that "racial prejudice" was a serious mental illness.

It was absolutely amazing to her how people could openly practice racism, lynch innocent folks, and yet claim to like the people that they mis-treat.

Whenever she heard some poor white man make a statement like:…"*hell, I ain't prejudice—I love these darkies…*" Melina knew that people like this were mentally warped souls, who desperately needed treatment. White people were just sick with the belief in "*White supremacy.*"

All her life she had experienced the phenomena that she had great insight and was somewhat clairvoyant. She knew from the time she was in elementary school that she was different from other kids, but did not know exactly why.

Melina's thoughts often flashed back to events in her life that had significantly effected her….such as her father's experiences in the military—

Nearly every Christmas and Thanksgiving, her family would go to their grandparents big house on Macedonia Ave. Her grandfather would tell stories of his ancestors, about slavery and other tales about his history. He often told the same story over and over about how his grandfather ran away from a plantation and lived with some Indians.

The Indians (native Americans) were very helpful to the Black slaves who escaped…and often took them into the tribes and married with them. His grandfather had married an Indian woman, who was a self-made herbalist, who practiced *"healing secrets"* that she had learned from her ancestors. It was one of his favorite dinner table topics.

Native American Indians knew a lot about using herbal remedies, spiritual rituals and mediation for healing. They also were deeply involved with concepts of *"taking care of nature and the Earth."* He often told stories of how their religious and spiritual beliefs would not permit them to participate in the enslavement of Black people that was occurring all around them in America.

Melina became very curious about these topics because of her grandfather's stories. She was even more curious about the herbs that were used to heal.

Melina was a student who loved to learn. She started studying about African-American slaves, black history, and topics like this on her own from books that she got from the public library. Nearly every Saturday a "bookmobile" came through their neighborhood—and Melina always checked out books to read.

She read comic books and many types of books on every topic that she could find—but most enjoyed learning about black history and her ancestors.

SCHOOL DAYS:

Melina began Kindergarten at Bigfellow Elementary School. She did very well and when she reached the 2nd grade, her teacher informed her parents that Melina was extremely bright and could write stories.

As she grew up in a small Black ghetto-type community in Indiana, she found that she did very well in school—in fact, her grades were often all "A's" and a few "B's"—which made some of the other kids jealous. On report card day, she found herself hiding her grades and running home to keep from getting into a fight with one of the cruel kids.

While the other elementary school students were struggling to be able to produce a decent sentence, Melina was writing complete stories. Most of her teachers were amazed with her abilities.

All through-out Elementary and Junior High School, Melina demonstrated that she had a high degree of intelligence and a wonderful gift of being able to express herself in writing. Her 5th grade teacher Mr. Garingo, who was one of her most favorite teachers, taught her how to play chess. One summer Melina entered into the City Wide Chess Tournament and won 2nd place.

Sometimes, she and her friends would ride on their bikes to the river and spend nearly all day there, listening to a radio, snacking and talking. The attraction of being directly in contact with plants, water, fish, nature, greenery, and sunshine was very pleasurable. In fact, it was a great escape from the harsh realities that they faced in a cold-hearted society.

One day when Melina was about 14 years old, she was there on the river bank with her sister, brother and father Melanin—when several loud-mouth rednecks drove up to them in a small raggedy pick-up truck. One of the white men yelled in a sarcastic tone,…*"Did you niggers catch anything today?"*

Well, Melanin was not in the mood for this crap…so he pulled out a small deringer that he kept in his belt and shot in the air above the white men's heads. They scattered like roaches when they saw the gun. Melanin shouted back at them…*"catch this!!!"* They were very accustomed to being harassed and ridiculed by white people in Middletown.

These were the times of racial segregation and harsh racial injustices. In those days there was blatant racial discrimination. Because of discrimination, these"minority groups" did not have open access to health care clinics, to hospitals or to other health services. Non-white people were relegated to find whatever health care they could—or left to be treated by any ol' doctor that would treat them, whether he had a real license or not.

It was the worst of times. It was the best of times. It was the best of times because living was simple, easy and inexpensive. But it was also the worst of times, because there were a lot of social, health and political problems. Melina was very young when she learned that her mother's real mother had died of an illness while in childbirth. Doctors did not know what to do for her condition. She was always saddened by these thoughts.

She began keeping a diary of real-life events. Melina possessed special gifts for writing and telling stories. Some people thought she was just really smart. And others thought she was from another planet, because of her unusual insights, high level of intelligence and excellent language skills. In the minds of white folks—it was just unheard of in those days for a *"colored girl"* to have such abilities.

In fact, the teachers sent Melina to a psychologist at *Abnormal College* for testing. Melina made such a grand impression and high scores that she was promoted 2 grades higher.

When Melina was ready to enter the 9th grade, the Community Schools had constructed a brand new building. The new school was named Keener Jr. High School and it was situated on the border of the segregated *White and Black areas.* The White people in those areas were very upset with the thought that Black kids would be also permitted to go to that school.

Eventually, White people began threatening the Blacks, throwing rocks at them, spitting on them and burning crosses. The neighborhood was in an uproar for the entire first month that the new school was open.

During the first few days of school at Keener, Melina and her friends had to have police escorts and protection from the National Guard to be able to simply walk into the school. Why?…because many of the wonderful White folks in Middletown did not want any Black students to sit next to their precious White kids in a school. Melina's thoughts drifted back into some of the experiences that she had recorded in her diary….

STORIES FROM Melina's DIARY….

Every day for several months there was a big scene of mobs of White people protesting us outside the new school. They spit at us, yelled ugly names, and stood in crowds around the school building trying to intimidate the black kids who were coming to school. We had the sheriff and National Guard there to protect us for several weeks for the opening of the new school.

As I walked up the guarded sidewalk into the school building, I could hear the voices of White people yelling ugly profanities at the small group of Black students being escorted into the school.

During my year in 9th grade at Keener…there were many incidents of racial discrimination, harassment, and general hostility between Black folks and White folks.

Often times, the White students would pass by and spit on Black students as they rode their school buses home. The Blacks had to walk on a dusty road home.

Sometimes the Black students would retaliate by throwing rocks at the buses. I personally was one of the more active rock-throwers among my peers.

Even after some of this type of harassment calmed down, we continued to experience racial hostility. Nearly every week there was at least one major incident where white students yelled racial slurs at black students.

Months later, the teachers decided that we could have a *"Record Hop"*(dance) in the school cafeteria after school on a Friday—which hopefully would help us to make better relationships. Most of the students—black and white—were there. They played mostly "white music." This may have been because older white people claimed that *"Negro music was wild and savage."*

One of the black students asked them to play some of the popular black records—and so the DJ played "The Twist" by Chubby Checker. A crowd of students gathered in the middle of the cafeteria floor to watch some of us doing the new dance craze. Eventually the entire group—blacks and whites—were all twisting together.

Suddenly, a white teacher stopped the music. He told us all that *"it was not right for colored and white to dance together."* And then they shut down the Record Hop and sent us all home. My God!! We were not even touching each other.

****

SISTERHOOD:

Melina had many girlfriends who formed a club…which they called *"the Chain Gang."* They did things such as held car washes to raise money. Often they had slumber parties. This club was something that created a sisterhood for these little girls…a wonderful comraderie developed between them that has lasted forever. They developed pride and high self-esteem. They went fishing together, cooked and baked recipes, talked about boys, held birthday parties, and were just like sisters to each other for many years. It was a sisterhood.

And they often fought like a team against any White person who called them ugly names as they walked home from school. Getting harassed when walking home was common and these girls always stayed together for protection and self-preservation.

Every summer, 2 other girls (Deena & Rose) from Toledo used to visit their grandmother who lived in Brownly…nearly 6 blocks from Melina's house. Melina and her sister Karo and 2 girls from Toledo— were the best of friends.

During Melina's summer prior to entering high school, they all decided that they wanted to attend summer school together at Bunion School. Well, Bunion was out in the high class White community near Abnormal College…so these 4 girls would have to ride the bus or walk a long way. But they thought it would be fun, so they did.

One day as they walked together from summer school, they decided to stop to get ice cream at a little wooden building (stand) that was located on the bridge *(which connected Brownly to the rest of town)*.

The 4 girls walked peacefully up to the window to place their orders. There was an old crinkled woman inside who made ugly faces at the girls.

STORIES FROM Melina's DIARY….

We walked up the window at the Ice Cream parlor.
The old ugly white woman asked,
" Well, what do you want?"

So Rose answered, *"We want some ice cream. Don't you sell ice cream here? I want a malt and my sisters want something too.."*

Then I ordered my favorite…butter pecan. And the other girls stated their orders. Karo ordered a hot dog and coke, also.

The old woman put the orders just barely outside the little service window and took our money. Then this mean old witch reached outside the window and pushed the hot dog and coke onto the gravel and dirt. And then she shouted, *"You nig-gers take that and get on back across that bridge where you belong!!!"*

I was furious!!....and I asked Rose...
"Did you see that?? Did you hear what she called us?"

Suddenly the old woman yelled again...*" You darkies get out of here! Go back across the bridge where you belong."*

I snapped!!!—lost my cool and punched my fist through the little service window. I really tried hard to grab the old woman by the collar, but the woman jumped back. Then, Rose and Deena ran around to the rear of the building to try to get in through the back door.

We were angry and shouting...*"You poor white trash ...give us our money back! Who in the devil do you think you are??"*

But another old White woman managed to slam the back door and lock it before they could get inside. After 20 minutes of yelling, a police car suddenly drove up into the parking lot. The appearance of the police was no surprise to us, because it seemed that White folks always used the police to uphold their wrongs.

After talking to all of us for 10 min.—this big White officer managed to get a refund from the old women. Then he drove us little colored girls home.
Rose and I *(being the oldest daughters)* explained this mess to our parents. This was nothing new for us. Almost every

week we had to explain why we were arguing and fighting with some White folks in Middletown.

****

Middletown's Mayor had been the GRAND DRAGON of the KKK during the days when Melanin was in the military. Middletown had been the scene of many terrible racial incidents, including one that involved a lynching in nearby Munkee, Indiana. Melanin's father had found out that the KKK had lynched some black men about 25 miles outside of Middletown—and he rounded up several men from his church and they rode out there and cut the bodies down. They brought the bodies to their little church in Middletown.

When the KKK found out what these Black men had done—they rode to Middletown and surrounded the little one-room black church. The Black men involved all took their guns to the church and there was a "stand-off."

The only thing that kept this incident from turning into a major blood-bath was that the Sheriff and the Police stopped it and ran the KKK out of Middletown.

Melina recalls this incident clearly because her grandfather had obtained photos of the men as they hung from the ropes….and gave her a copy of the pictures. Many people talked about this lynching.

Melina was the oldest daughter who was the "egg-head" of the family. She had been very smart in school and loved books. She had also been active in the Civil Rights Movement and similar activities. Melina had been the only child that finished several college degrees, had been a teacher and corporate training manager. She had dreams of becoming a professional author.

Karo was 2 years younger than she and was the exact opposite type of person. Karo was wild and like to run the streets. Abby was the baby of the family and was a very talented fashion designer. Juan was the only boy—and he was a computer programmer.

While listening to her father's interview, Melina recalled many memories of her own about racial hostility and segregation. In fact, Melina had been keeping a recorded diary of these incidents since she was in Junior High School. By the time she graduated from Middletown Central High School, her diary was full and she started keeping a Journal.

She had fond memories of the times when she was in high school and she and her friends would take rides out into the äll-White neighborhoods to find the little statues of the Negro jockeys—the "coon symbols"—and such—so that they could destroy them. Hunting these little statues was a lot of fun—but the most fun was taking a bat and busting them up and then escaping from the scene before anyone knew who did it.

Each time that she experienced any form of harassment, mis-treatment, or racism—Melina wrote about it in her JOURNAL. She called her Journal: *"Slave Ship Records: The African Hell-a-cost."*

She kept this Journal because she never wanted anyone to have any amnesia about this history of these racist events. She had realized at a young age that many people want to cover up the social problems and pretend that slavery was a good thing. This Journal was an antedote against people who easily develop "historical amnesia" and want to pretend that the terrible acts of racism, lynchings, harassment, and other insulting events never happened. One day she hoped to publish these stories.

Back in those days, there were very few published Black American authors—and in high school, her counselor told her—*"you should try to choose a more practical career for a colored girl..."*—but Melina had made a commitment to one day write books on these topics. Melina thought that the counselor was nothing but another racist white lady who wanted to see Negroes in subservient degrading positions.

After she graduated from high school, Melina enrolled in the college right there in Middletown——Abnormal State University. When she started taking classes, she learned that the professors, staff and other officials of the college were also very racist and that "white supremacy " was alive and well.

In one of her English classes, the students were given the assignment to write a story about something significant that happened when they were young which changed their life drastically. So, Melina used one of the stories from her Journal:

AN INCIDENT THAT CHANGED MY LIFE:

When I was approximately 12 years old my sister and brother and I loved to go to the movies. The Ravioli Theatre often had specials on Saturdays when they showed 6 or 8 features of cartoons, cowboys, and "3 Stooges." It only cost 25 cents admission—for all of the shows.

One cold Saturday in December when we were all out of school for vacation break, we asked our mother if we could go to the Ravioli Theatre. She piled us up in the car and drove us there. There were hundreds of kids lined up to get into the show.

My mother told us to call her when it was over so that she could give us a ride. She did not want us walking in that cold weather.

So, my sister and brother and I went in and sat in the balcony—where the colored people were forced to sit. After 5 hours of movies—it was all over. Black and white kids were lined up at the pay phones trying to call for their parents because the weather had turned colder and it was snowing heavily outside.

I decided to go next door to the restaurant to use the pay phone there—hoping to get around waiting in that long line in the theatre.

When we walked up to the door of the restaurant—a huge white man stood in front of us—as if to block us from coming in. He asked me, *"Now just what do you darkies want?"*

I informed him that I simply wanted to use the phone to call my mother. He responded with—*"We do not allow darkies in here."* Then he slammed the door in our faces.

So—there I was, downtown with my younger brother and sister, in the cold snow—and not much chance of getting to a phone quickly. We went to down the block to another store—where I could see a pay phone through the window.
When we walked in—the white clerk suddenly stopped what she was doing and asked me—"Now what do you want?"

"I just want to use the pay phone…" I told her.

To which she responded—*" Well, this phone is out of order. So go someplace else."*

We left—and as I got outside the store—I looked back in through the window and watched another white woman pick up the receiver on the pay phone and use it to make a call.

Finally, I decided to drag my sister and brother through the cold blizzard to the Police Station. It was a long walk—but we got there OK. A kind white policeman gladly called my mother to come and get us.

I was extremely hurt, angry and upset. I wanted to burn this business down. I hated white folks for their actions like this. I wanted to just make them all leave Planet Earth!!!

This incident changed the way I viewed society and caused me to make a commitment to fight for justice.
I was not allowed to be "innocent and happy" like the little white children.

This was an event that significantly altered my life because it represented many other similar terrible , painful incidents that I experienced—
WHILE GROWING UP BLACK.
****

Melina turned in her typed up paper and got an "A" from the professor. The professor wrote a note on it and said—
- *"you are an excellent story teller and insightful writer."*

Because of these incidents with racism and segregation Melina became much more vocal and started speaking out against white racism, injustices and segregation. Little did she realize at that time——Melina's Journal would eventually be used to tell stories about these racists incidents all over the United States—and perhaps the world.

She recalled that she took part in many of the Civil Rights protest marches and rallies back in the 1950' s and all thru the 1960's and

1970's. Growing up Black was a very unique experience—and needed to be recorded, she believed.

Melina returned her attention to her father's interview after reminiscing about her own experiences as a Black American female. Her father was now talking about how segregation and discrimination had harmed all black people and forced them to live on the brink of self-destruction in poverty.

These types of racial incidents permeated Melina's life as a Black person growing up in Middletown USA. This is the information that is missing from the other books and studies done about MIDDLETOWN AMERICA.

===

NOTE: If you would like to read more of these stories about Melina's life,—Get a copy of the book:

Middletown Roots
—by Melvia Miller

===

COLLECTIBLE VALUABLE INFO—#11

"MONEY TALKS—
Creating Wealth"

"There is no security on this Earth…only Opportunities."
~ Douglas MacArthur

INTRODUCTION:

Many of the terrible ordeals, wars and social problems of the past were rooted in the need for money and survival. Of course, we cannot survive without some type of economy—but history has not shown a pretty picture when it comes to mankind's attempts to create a healthy-wealthy economic system that benefits most of its citizens. From the beginning of human civilization—the issue of providing food, clothing and shelter—for most of this Earth's citizens—have been a chronic unsolved problem.

Hunger and poverty still continue to haunt most of the world—even into the 21st Century. Sickness and early death are rampant in many "under-developed" countries. These horrible conditions did not happen by accident. Africa is not in the pits of despair and poverty by accident or because of "inferiority" of its people. The poverty and suffering that causes thousands of Mexicans to risk their lives crossing the border—did not develop by accident either. Politicians, leaders, and gangsters have all had a hand in creating the poor economic situation of the world.

The problems in the economic arena manifested because people became greedy and ruthless, and thus created economic systems that were harmful, unjust, cruel, and unbalanced. They began to exploit workers, to cheat women out of equal pay, to discriminate against Blacks and other minority group workers—*and much worse*

American history is marred by the battles and disputes between the workers and management.

All throughout the history of the USA there have been corrupt business practices, exploitation of labor, and other unscrupulous ways used to make money—including the Mafia, gangs, prostitution, illegal drug trafficking, and worse!

Child-labor has been used in some countries in order to get away with paying small wages to innocent children and to get the most work for little pay. Prostitution has been a way of exploiting women for monetary gain. Women who participate in this system do not gain much— and many die terrible deaths at a young age.

The African Slave Trade had one ultimate goal—which was to enrich the slave-owners and promote the plantation economy. FREE SLAVE LABOR provided most of the basis for the progress and success of the United States economy before the 1900's.

Before the 1940's most people *(approx. 80% of the U.S. population)* operated their own small business…such as farming, local stores, barber shops, repair shops, beauty salons, tailor shops, janitorial services, etc.

During the *Industrial Revolution* period, machinery was widely used to make products and companies learned to manufacture products by using assembly line workers. People worked long hours for minimum wages producing goods that would eventually be sold in retail stores for great profits for the manufacturers.

Our nation grew to become a country filled with huge corporations—and 90% of the work-force had jobs with these big companies. The major World Wars also brought about changes in the way Americans worked and lived.

Huge corporations grew from this type of economy——only to find themselves suffering in a down-turn. The employees were subject to any and all rules laid down by the management—while the management reaped most of the benefits, profits, and good returns from the corporations.

Millions of workers found themselves subjected to financial trouble simultaneously when the corporations are not doing well.

Although our Federal and State governments have attempted to offer "affordable housing" programs and other services—many people still remain in sub-standard housing or homeless… and many senior citizens live on tiny budgets after working most of their lives——while simultaneously others in this nation live in big mansions and huge homes, and have exorbitant amounts of wealth and use their money for blatant foolishness.

The existence of widespread homelessness in the richest country in the world is a very pathetic indicator of our nation's priorities. In many cities, people who have regular jobs—earning $12.00 to $25.00 per hour—cannot afford decent homes!

What does it profit a society to gain power and riches—if it loses its own soul???

In countries like Afghanistan—the wealthy terrorists who made money from sales of drugs and other under-handed ways—failed to use that money to develop a good economy for the citizens of their own nation. Afghanistan is one of the poorest nations in the world….and their dictator leaders (the Taliban) foolishly think that they can perpetrate their exploitations upon other nations.

In the 21st Century—people in the inner cities in the richest country in the world (USA) still suffer from hunger, homelessness, poverty, lack of training, sickness and other ailments—directly related to a poor economic system. Many people who work regular jobs cannot find affordable decent housing and live in "shelters" or in other sub-standard conditions.

After many centuries of societies struggling for ways to feed its population, to provide for its citizens the basics of FOOD, CLOTHING AND SHELTER, and to establish decent housing, schools, clinics, hospitals, stores, and businesses—We have learned many lessons upon which we can begin to build a new type of economy—one that is not harmful to other people, one that does not put others in slavery, and one that is compatible with creating a good ecology.

The world has changed and so must the way we do business and make money. Success must be measured in a different and more humane way.

It seems that America is the richest country in the world in terms of materialism—but extremely poor in other areas—such as in spiritual values, morality and a sense of compassion for the less fortunate.

In recent years—thousands of people have left the work-force and started their own successful home-based businesses.

STEPS TO SUCCESS:

"The man who will use his skill and constructive imagination to see how much he can give for a dollar...instead of how much he can get for a dollar is bound to succeed."

~ Henry Ford *(auto tycoon)*

STEP # 1—VISUALIZE what you want....—

- Do you want some new furniture?
- Do you want that new car?
- Would you like to take a trip to Hawaii?
- Or would you like to have more free time?
- A better, safer community?
- Discounts on medical & dental care?
- To become a published author?

Whatever it is that you dream of—visualize it. Cut out pictures of the car, house, clothing—and other items that you want. Keep them in a scrap-book so that you can look at them from time to time.

In the modern times of computers, the Internet, CD burners, DVD players, and laser printers, a new form of economy has come to the forefront—known as:

HOME BASED BUSINESSES.

All new inventions, new technology, new best-selling books, and other creations began with a dream—a vision of what it may look like and what benefit it might serve. So dream !!

STEP #2—Research methods and resources for achieving what you want....

Then begin to take action by researching various ways to make your dreams come true. Write down some weekly goals of things you want to accomplish in order to work toward your larger goals.

Millions of people are now learning to make money from the comfort of their homes by advertising, selling and marketing

their own unique products and services via the use of the Internet, classified ads, networking, and other ways of promotion. Some home-based entrepreneurs are making thousands of dollars each month in businesses, such as:
REAL ESTATE, MLM sales, Advertising agencies, product sales, music, mail order, Consulting Services, Speaker's Services, and DESK-TOP PUBLISHING.

Home-based businesses do not require large offices, lots of employees, extensive record-keeping, workman's compensation insurance, or many of the other over-head expenses of the typical retail shops that have been popular in the past. Most of the people who have made it big—started very small.

BELIEVE IT OR NOT—in the past 20 years, more millionaires have been created in 4 major types of home-based businesses which began at home on a low budget—

(1)Multi-level Marketing
(MLM—Network Marketing)
and Mail Order Sales
and
2) Computer/Internet Services
and
3) Real Estate sales & services
and
4)The Hip-Hop (Rap) Music business.

Businesses such as"*Mary Kay Cosmetics,*"... "*Nature's Sunshine—health products*"..."*Amway*"... and "*Pre-paid Legal Svcs.*" are the type of home-based or small businesses *(or MLM business)* which have created many millionaires. There are many of these MLM-type businesses that are thriving. Participants benefit by helping others to become successful.

Mail Order Sales are often used in conjunction with other programs which permit entrepreneurs to purchase products at low discounts and to re-sell them at a profit.

Sears & Roebuck got started back in the 1940's with a printed mail order catalog and became some of the first mail order millionaires Most successful businesses utilize some form of MAIL ORDER in order to reach the widest base of customers.

SUCCESS STORIES:

Bill Gates found a way to create technology that many people want and use. He became the Microsoft billionaire. The WWF Wrestler "Rock"—was sleeping on a dirty mattress when he started promoting himself as a WWF wrestler. Now he is living "large."

And then there is the success story of Whoopie Goldberg and Poetess Maya Angelou—both of whom started at very low points in life and rose to the top.

Oprah Winfrey found a niche in the "Talk TV Show" business…but she started very small on a local channel in Chicago. She learned the keys to marketing her show and now enjoys the benefits. Jerry Springer managed to corner another market in that same arena and make millions of dollars.

The "Rap Music" business did more to generate wealth than did all the "food stamp programs" CETA and "wars on poverty" and welfare programs ever created by the government. "Master P"—One of the most popular "rap artists" who is a self-made millionaire began his business out of his home by burning his own CDs and selling them on consignment in local neighborhood stores. He is now a multi-millionaire. Other "rap star millionaires" include: SNOOP DOGGY DOGG, DR. DRE, and WILL SMITH.

STEP # 3—Learn what works and the keys for making a lot of money….. find out what kinds of products sell or systems & programs or plans work !

KEYS TO MAKING MONEY:

The main key to making these types of business work is to find a system that creates a "win-win" situation for both the client and the business owners. Wealth is created by marketing a valuable product or service that fulfills and need or desire to mass numbers of people.
MARKET SOMETHING THAT PEOPLE WANT ENJOY, AND DESIRE—something that helps other people….and you will meet with success.

ARE YOU TIRED OF THE "40-40-40-40 PLAN"??

You know…the one where you work 40 hrs.
per week for 40 years—and pay 40% in tax
—only to retire at a 40% reduced income…..

DO YOU FIND THAT YOU HAVE MORE MONTH LEFT OVER THAN MONEY?

OR PERHAPS YOU ARE SICK & TIRED OF YOUR DEAD-END JOB.....

WOULD YOU LIKE TO HAVE MORE MONEY TO ENJOY LIFE...
(buy a new car, new house, new furniture,
new clothes, & take a vacation)?

HOW ABOUT FINDING MONEY IN YOUR MAILBOX???

—WOULD THAT BE SOMETHING THAT WOULD ENHANCE YOUR LIFE?

CHANGE YOUR MIND...
IMPROVE YOUR INCOME...

TO BECOME FINANCIALLY INDEPENDENT or RICH...WE MUST START WITH A SOLID PLAN.

Not long ago our country was run by small businesses—home-based operations that served the needs of their communities. Approximately 60 years ago,more than 75% of the businesses were small—people owned their own enterprises....and the rest were large corporations which hired employees.When the majority of people owned their own business, there was not a widespread fear of being laid off.

After going through a 60 year period of forming major companies, giant corporations, and huge stores, we now find that the need for services offered by the small business has increased more than ever.Too many people are waiting for that *"big dream job"* to come along. They often ignore the signs of a sluggish economy, avoid any thoughts of starting their own business, and suffer in "dead-end, low-paying" jobs. Many of these same people will IGNORE opportunities to make money from their own business—and turn their noses up at any and all "home-based businesses."

Many people are 'broke' or in financial trouble because they waste the money they do have or they live far above their means.

Many Americans are deep in debt with credit cards and loans…but have only a few material things to show for it all.

If you are serious about changing your financial status—you must begin now!!

CHANGE YOUR THINKING ABOUT MONEY !

If you are spending more than you can afford…using means such as: credit
cards, loans, and gambling—that is the root cause of your financial problems.

Analyze what you do with your money every week. Are you spending most of it on foolishness, wine, women and song, on entertainment, on clothing, on sports—or on just plain junk???
Are your expenditures really benefiting you ?
Or are you investing some and saving some?
Are you using your money to promote your business?

BEGIN RIGHT WHERE YOU ARE TODAY…. START WITH A PLAN FOR SAVING….QUIT LIVING on the edge—*ON CREDIT*—from paycheck to paycheck—

ANYONE CAN CHANGE THEIR INCOME BY DOING THE RIGHT THINGS TO ACHIEVE THEIR GOALS.

There are numerous books on the market and at the public library that are filled with ideas, resources, places to obtain low cost products, marketing techniques—and even FREE STUFF, free government grants—and everything you need to know to make money from home.

BEGIN BY READING SOME OF THESE BOOKS.

You are invited to join the *"Quiet Revolution"*——

MAKING MONEY FROM YOUR OWN HOME BASED BUSINESS…..

ONE OF THE BEST WAYS TO START ON A SMALL BUDGET FROM HOME IS IN THE MAIL ORDER BUSINESS….

If you have been seeking a way to increase your income, and have more free time to travel and enjoy life—then MAIL ORDER MARKETING may be the answer to what you have been seeking.

The Mail Order business has been around as far back as the days of the establishment of the first post offices. Mail Order sales have been profitable for many years—as far back as when Sears & Roebuck first published and distributed their product catalogs.

Mail Order techniques are used by the large corporations, by the U.S. Government, by Health Agencies and by small businesses as a way to advertise and promote their services and products to huge numbers of people.

And by using small ads, many people in home-based businesses have created huge incomes via the use of the mail.

Many people go to college and study courses that help them to improve their skills in subjects such as English, Spanish, Math, Science and History. Most people go to college in hopes of being able to have a better job, make more money and enjoy life.

Unfortunately, in this economy which has become less dependent upon workers and more technologically based——even many people with college degrees are not satisfied with their income, find themselves in debt, or simply are over-worked and have little time to enjoy their families and travel.

When people study courses that are offered in the schools and colleges across the USA they expect a return in terms of better employment, improvement of skills—or something of value. Unfortunately there are very few courses that actually teach a step-by-step method up the ladder to the wealth. There are only a few good courses available on the subject of *'how to enhance your income in a small business or from a home-based business.'*

BENEFITS OF HOME-BASED BUSINESSES:

And there are many advantages to having your own business. If you keep good records and set yourself up as a legitimate business, you can deduct most of your costs for business from your taxes.

Did you know that there are basically 2 tax systems in this country? ONE system is for the business owner. The other system is designed for the workers. Workers simply pay certain taxes and have few benefits and allowances.

However, the U.S. Government has established many opportunities, tax advantages and other incentives for small businesses. A small business can deduct the costs of advertising, inventory, office supplies, travel, vehicle expenses, printing, postage, computers, and much more….and cut back on the amount of taxes paid.

THE IDEAL HOME-BASED BUSINESS:

MAIL ORDER MARKETING is very lucrative because the potential customer base is broad and vast. A good printed sales catalog or sales letter has the potential of reaching thousands or millions of people in all areas of the world. In the Mail Order business, entrepreneurs are not limited to the few customers who may visit their store-front or office. In Mail Order….the businessperson's market is opened up to millions of potential customers.

Mail Order techniques allow the entrepreneur to reach a wide range of potential customers via classified ads, mailers, post cards, and other avenues.

By using mail order to advertise, the business-person is not limited to the few people in the neighborhood who might purchase something….but instead increases his market to a broad base of people who see the ads.   And if you join your business with a good "network marketing" company/service/product—you can easily realize a greater income.

In other words, if you are already selling a product via an MLM company (such as *Shaklee, Amway, Excell, Pre-Paid Legal Service,* or something similar)—you can greatly improve your income and prospects by utilizing MAIL ORDER TECHNIQUES.

Mail Order businesses are multi-million dollar enterprises. Many millionaires have made their fortunes via mail order. With a desirable product/service and ways to advertise, almost anyone can create a good business by mail.

You have probably seen people on TV talking about how they made lots of money by selling something by mail. However, you probably did not get any information on how they got started in this business. You may have also seen the sales letters that make claims of "creating millionaires."

In order to be successful in mail order, one must have the goal of building a business and a customer base. There is more to becoming successful in this enterprise than just randomly mailing out some flyers. There are actually techniques that have been tested by many mail order entrepreneurs that work. Don't try to re-invent the wheel—but instead learn what has already proven to work.

KEYS TO BUSINESS SUCCESS:

Offer something of value to your customers!

...DISCOUNTS, FREE STUFF, COUPONS, FREE RESOURCES, etc.

CREATIVE ADVERTISING, OFFERING FREE GIFTS AND DISCOUNTS—AND SELLING A PRODUCT OR SERVICE THAT IS BENEFICIAL TO CONSUMERS—WILL LEAD YOU TO SUCCESS.

What do people want and need?

- *Good health & fitness*
- *Discounts and savings*
- *To be more efficient, safe and happy.*
- *Sources for making money*
- *Weight loss*
- *Improved lifestyle*

The people who have made lots of money in mail order have found that there are certain "keys" to success. They have been able to make those *"keys"* work for their benefit. Most of us have received some type of brochure, advertisement, sales letter or catalog by mail which invites us to buy something, join something, or participate in something.

The people who mail out these materials are most likely using some of the techniques and steps involved in developing a good mail order business. Although there are many deceptive mailer programs out there—there are also many legitimate companies that utilize mail order and earn huge profits, such as *Walter Drake (stationery)*.

One "key" to getting responses is to offer some type of valuable benefit to your potential customer—perhaps a FREE GIFT....or some other incentive for their participation. The word: "Free" always attracts attention and potential customers.

Another "Key" to your small business success is to create brochures, flyers and other advertising that is easy to read and that contains an ORDER FORM to make it easy for the customer to order the product. If the customers have to compose their own 'ordering forms' or type long letters to respond to get info from you—they will tend to not do it. MAKE IT EASY TO ORDER YOUR PRODUCTS. The less *"work"* you put on the customer, the better your reception will be.

ANOTHER KEY—

Networking with other up-scale business people is one key ingredient to improving your business ventures. Networking means meeting people, communicating with others, and building a group of supporters, clients, and resources for your business.

If you are a doctor, lawyer, hair-dresser, mechanic, writer, or musician that is operating a business—networking is essential to increasing your span of operation.

Networking is a concept that involves getting the word out about whatever services or products you offer—and meeting people who may be of assistance or who may become customers.

When you attend conferences, meetings, or join clubs—get out and talk to people, give them your business cards, flyers and e-mail address.

Even if you are doing MAIL ORDER marketing, your ads, announcements, offers, and brochures need to find their way into the hands of customers.

A FUNNY THING HAPPENS WHEN WE DO NOT COMMUNICATE OR ADVERTISE…nothing.

It is a rare and unusual business that can simply sit quietly—never promote or place an ad—and /or make money without advertising and networking with other people.

Many small businesses fail each year because they DO NOT ADVERTISE!!!!!

For some odd reason, many small business owners have the mis-conception that they only need to "open up shop" with a few products—and the clients will stampede into their business.

In any business endeavor, we must understand the value and importance of creating good relationships with customers, suppliers, clients and others with whom we become involved.

TEST MARKETING:

Before investing thousands of dollars in a big ad campaign—run small inexpensive ads to "test' the response. Use the least expensive classified ads that have the longest run times. Some publications are *"weekly"* or *"monthly"*
editions—that give maximum exposure to your ad. Start with those.

Try your ad in different types of papers, in newsletters, in the Church Bulletin, in the local college papers, in free magazines, on the Internet— *(and so on)*—

and then track the responses in order to determine who is responding, which ad is the most effective and what works for your offers.

USE CREATIVITY to find your customers !

Track your ads by coding them in some way so that you know which source is producing the most responses. STOP running ads that do not produce. And run more of the ones that are getting responses.

In conducting mail order, keep in mind that only a small percentage of people are going to respond to any advertisement. And from those responses, only another small percentage is going to purchase something. If you are simply looking to sign up in a good home-based, business, usually the best opportunities are in those that use "Multi-level marketing" structures.

WHAT IS NETWORK MARKETING—???

'MLM'—aka: 'Multi-Level Marketing'
also known as: "NETWORK MARKETING"—
is a method of direct sales of goods &
services & products…using independent

distributors who promote said products,
sign up\sponsor other distributors and
make customer referrals.

This revolutionary business concept has created
thousands of wealthy home-based entrepreneurs
in the past 30 years—many of whom earn over
$30,000 per year from working at home.

Many thousands of people have left the 'rat-race' of their hectic jobs, and started doing business from home—by mail, over the Internet, and using MLM -type companies. Some earn several thousand dollars each month from home. To be successful in any business, you must research to find the best products at the lowest prices, and/or the unique services that you can offer to your customers and clients.

One of the best ways to start out is to get involved with a solid MLM (*multi-level marketing or network marketing*) company. Why? Because the good ones have already established their services, goods, products and ways to advertise.

By joining a good MLM program, the products, advertising brochures, and most of what you need to operate a business will be provided. And most of these MLM companies offer excellent pay and rewards for their distributors.

There are many of these types of companies, so take time to go to their *"opportunity meetings"* and find the one that best suits your needs and desires.

And in MLM businesses, people help each other to become successful. The more your help the others who join your group—the more money you make. In a good MLM business—it is a WIN-WIN situation for all involved.

BASIC ASPECTS of Network Marketing:

MLM is also known as 'Network Marketing' because it includes the building of a network of distributors who advertise the company's products…using person-to-person contact. MLM offers the chance to earn money from the efforts of other people. By building a group of reps who help each other to win—everyone can succeed.

Also, these MLM companies are able to offer customers an opportunity to join as an independent distributor/rep and thus have their own home-based business.

WHEN IS THE LAST TIME YOU TOLD
SOMEONE ABOUT A GOOD MOVIE OR A
GOOD RESTAURANT or ANOTHER GOOD SERVICE ???

*When your referral went there and
purchased something, did that theatre
or restaurant send you a commission
for referring your associate to them?
Probably Not.

BUT THIS IS THE CONCEPT ON WHICH
"network marketing" THRIVES….
(referrals & word-of-mouth advertising)—
Many traditional corporations & businesses
are transferring their old methods of
direct retail selling to include some
forms of MLM (network marketing).

***COMPANIES SUCH AS—
Gillette, Avon, Mary Kay Cosmetics,
Rexall, Unidial, IBM, Coca-Cola,
General Motors, Amway, Tupperware, Pre-paid Legal Services, Ameri-Plan,
(and many others)—
are now using MLM (networking) methods.

WHY??
Because it one of the most powerful, profitable
business concepts to have ever existed…and
everyone benefits.

The term *"multi-level"* refers to the pay plan.
MLM Commissions are paid to distributors on
various levels of their organizations.
Each distributor benefits financially from
'over-rides' on the efforts of others' work.
This is how people build up huge incomes of
thousands of $$$ per month.

FOR EXAMPLE:

Mary recruits/sponsors Jerry.
Mary earns over-ride commissions
from Jerry's efforts.
Jerry recruits/sponsors Ellen.
Then both Mary & Jerry benefit from
Ellen's sales & recruiting.
And it goes on & on for many levels….

NOT ALL HOME-BASED (MLM) COMPANIES ARE THE SAME....

Each company has its own variation of a marketing plan that is based upon distributors (brokers, reps, agents) earning extra over-ride commissions from the efforts of other people in the business. Some companies have very solid programs and pay their reps very well.

And there are those that are not so good.

CHARACTERISTICS OF THE BEST
(MLM) 'NETWORKING' COMPANIES...

1) The better MLM companies offer bonuses, referral fees, gifts, & awards—such as: food coupons, car payments, or travel allowances. Pay plans should offer bonuses for those who 'go the extra mile'and produce a lot of business.

2) Good companies offer promotional assistance (such as professional, type-set brochures, flyers & postcards)& advertising help and leads, videos, recorded message hotlines,or other types of assistance in recruiting new distributors.

3) The better MLM companies have a web-site on the Internet. New customers can get information and/or sign up on-line, which opens the market to the whole world. Being on the Internet expands thepotential market for business to the entire world.

> ***Remember—there are many types of businesses and services that you can start with little or no start-up fees. There are hundreds of good companies that offer solid MLM plans.*

LOOK BEFORE YOU LEAP.
It all depends upon what you want.

4) START-UP COSTS:—Gauge the fees or investment for getting started
with the quality of what the company is offering....
* Are its present reps making money?
* Does the company provide a high-quality
'starter kit' filled with tools to do the business professionally?
* Are the present distributors successful?
* Research the background of the company.
* Is the company well-financed???

Good companies do not charge high fees simply
to get started (sign up). There are many
good MLM companies which have low start-up
costs—less than $100.—but yet offer a good program.

BEWARE if a company asks that distributors
buy & stock hundreds of products
in their homes to re-sell.

5) Good companies do not require that distributors urchase huge quan-
tities of products to deliver. A good company will ship directly to your
referred customer & then send you the commissions for making the
referrals. Or they will offer huge discounts to distributors for purchases.

****

HOW CAN COMPANIES AFFORD TO PAY THIS MUCH MONEY TO DISTRIBUTORS?

Very simple—instead of spending all or most of their funds on advertising in newspapers & TV, for salaries, etc.—they use that same money to pay distributors.

NETWORK MARKETING is a financial business concept/idea that has created thousands of millionaires in the past 30 years. It is a 'people-to-people' way of making loads of money.

IT IS LIKE HAVING A McDonald's Hamburger or Burger King FRAN-CHISE in your own home. Wealth and riches are created by mass marketing something. Just look at the world of entertainment, sports, publishing, recording arts, real estate or other sales.

MASS MARKETING IS THE SECRET:

How did people like Steven Speilberg, Michael Jackson, Oprah Winfrey or Bill Gates get rich?

It was not by working for someone else. They found their success by mass marketing something of value to huge numbers of people. You must be able to acquire a product at low cost—and re-sell it at a mark-up to thousands of customers.

WHY small HOME-BASED (MLM) BUSINESSES FAIL—

Many people have tried to make a fortune in their own home-based business….by selling lotions, potions, cleaners, soaps, cosmetics, or dog food. Unless you have managed to select the right products and to learn to do effective advertising, this also has been a major struggle for most people.

Many people who have experience in other MLM programs have found that they do not like the following aspects…

> a) Most of us do not like personal selling to friends OR tele-marketing.
> b) Over-priced products cause drop-outs.
> c) Stocking up on costly inventory.
> d) Hunting for new customers.
> e) Poor support from the company managers.
> f) Poor company compensation plan.

Unfortunately many thousands of people have tried to make money in MLMs and other *"programs"*—only to fail. Some people jump from company to company, from program to program—trying to find their fortune….chasing after empty promises of earning a huge income based upon someone *"fantastic compensation plan"*—or *"get rich quick scheme."*

INTERNET BUSINESSES:

And then let us not forget the crash of the hundreds of Internet businesses—the *"dot-coms"* that became—*"dot-bombs."*

Businesses on the Internet are also subject to the same influences, customer demands, economy, and environment as all other businesses.

Many of the companies that crashed on the Internet were not the small entrepreneurs doing simple mail order sales—rather they crashed because of "over-shooting their capability"——having major investors, high over-head expenses, lots of employees to support, big offices and poor planning.

Some of the entrepreneurs who invested in the "Internet boom" mistakenly thought that—because the Internet has world-wide customer base——that just offering anything on the Web would be a free ride to financial success. It does not work that easily.

Although the Internet is a fantastic marketing tool with broad appeal and mass out-reach—putting a business on the Internet still requires the same planning, surveying, and other techniques to promote such a business and acquire customers.

The Internet is a great source for finding products, services and opportunities. By using a "search engine"—it is possible to find all sorts of business opportunities, low cost products, resources for grants and loans, and much more.

HAVE A MILLION DOLLAR DAY!!

"Dictators in America"

FREE NEWS REPORT:

TRUTH is often stranger than FICTION....

"AMERICA'S BIGGEST BUSINESS RIP-OFF"

Our society has lived through all types of crises, difficulties, and upheaval...ranging from The Civil War to WW I and WWII to surviving the "cold war" with Russian communist threats and the Vietnam War. We found the cure for Polio and other serious diseases and managed to partially de-segregate the public schools. We have also struggled through the Civil Rights marches and protests of the 1960's and the 1970's and witnessed many improvements in our nation.

We are now facing another monumental problem that is not so obvious to many people, but nevertheless no less of a serious matter.

THIS HORRIBLE CANCER UPON OUR SOCIETY IS:
Bad faith insurance practices.

re: *HOT STORY:*
"The Horrible Social Problem of 'bad faith' insurance practices..."

AMERICANS ARE HAVING THEIR CIVIL AND CONSTITU-
TIONAL RIGHTS ARBITRARILY VIOLATED BY MAJOR CORRUPT
INSURANCE COMPANIES....AND ARE BEING UNFAIRLY AND
ILLEGALLY VICTIMIZED BY THIS INSURANCE AND HEALTH
CARE SYSTEM—A PROBLEM THAT WILL EVENTUALLY BRING
OUR SOCIETY TO A POINT OF REVOLT, REBELLION, PROTEST,
AND DESTRUCTION.

THE FOLLOWING REPORT IS RELEASED IN ORDER TO EXPOSE
THE TRUTH ABOUT MAJOR INSURANCE BAD FAITH ACTIONS....
FOR THE BENEFIT OF CONSUMERS AND ALL OTHERS WHO
HAVE BEEN EFFECTED BY THE TERRIBLE ACTIONS OF INSUR-
ANCE COMPANIES.

DESCRIPTION OF THE PROBLEM:

Bad faith insurance practices have grown rapidly and become a very
serious mainstream problem of epidemic proportions—threatening all
Americans. Until now, the only way for claimants, injured parties,
patients or policy-holders to fight the insurance companies or to collect
on an unfairly denied claim was to fight in Court.

Many people are fighting the illegal, corrupt and fraudulent actions
of major insurance companies who are using every dirty trick in the
book in order to evade payment of claims. Greedy major insurance
companies have been acting to the detriment of injured people,
patients, doctors, clinics and everyone involved.

EVEN THOUGH THE LAWS STATE THAT INSURANCE COMPA-
NIES MUST PROMPTLY EVALUATE AND SETTLE CLAIMS—this
law is violated, ignored or circumvented on a regular basis. Why?

Insurance companies gain HUGE PROFITS by denying claims. Approximately 95% of people who have claims denied do not fight back, even though they know they have been cheated. These victims walk away angry. Thus, leaving the insurance company to either go to arbitration or Court with perhaps only 5% (or less) of the people who file claims against them. In summary—BAD FAITH denial of claims is very profitable for the insurance companies.

First to blame is our legislature (SENATORS, CONGRESSMEN, REPS) and State Insurance Commissioners, politicians and insurance adjusters who have worked to permit these insurance companies to demand that consumers pay outrageous costs to simply have auto insurance or health insurance—and then to systematically deny payment of legitimate claims. The Insurance Companies have been very instrumental in getting laws passed that help them to virtually operate without any supervision or legal accountability.

There are laws to protect claimants, but most states do not uphold them well.

Hospitals, clinics, doctors, chiropractors, psychologists, therapists and others who have treated injured people have been unfairly denied payment of these medical bills. In far too many cases there are attorneys or insurance adjusters who are in essence practicing medicine without a license and making decision about the patient's treatment (or non-treatment.)

And to make the problem even worse, injured parties, consumers, patients, and the public have little recourse. We all have the option of hiring an attorney—who can then be bombarded and tied up in ridiculous arguments of medical reports—by the unethical actions of the attorneys and IMEs who work for the corrupt insurance companies.

And at the end of this road, patients, consumers and injured parties can file a lawsuit and take the matter to Court—before a JURY of "laymen"—who know little to nothing about medical issues, treatments, etc.

THE PATTERN OF BAD FAITH INSURANCE:

Insurance Companies send reps to lobby for them and go to the legislature, to Court, and campaign for the public to pay them higher premiums, that laws be passed that the public must purchase insurance to drive—and other acts that benefit these insurers financially.

Insurance companies are violating all sorts of regulations and laws that govern them—and the STATE INSURANCE COMMISSIONS do very little to stop these horrible practices.

HMO's and other Health Insurers are also involved in failing to pay legitimate claims. Many times these health insurers simply deny coverage for treatments that are seriously needed by patients or they deny payment for emergency treatments given by doctors. Many people have been on their "near-death bed"—only to have their health care insurance deny payment for much needed medication, doctor's care, therapy or treatments....for no legitimate reason.

Medical doctors, chiropractors, health care providers, clinics and other people who treat injured patients have been unfairly caught up in a system that requires them to treat injured people—without payment—based upon a "lien" against the accident claim. And then most doctors may wait from 2 to 6 years (or more) while the patient and attorneys have to fight insurance companies for payment.

And if that is not bad enough—the insurance companies then try every dirty trick in the book to "deny" the claim—to argue that the doctors "over-treated" the patient, or to even argue in Court that the injured party was not even hurt in the first place.

Many physicians and health care providers have been cheated out of payments due to them because of these ridiculous claims that insurance companies have made in Court. Any excuse that they can muster is used to take a case to court and put on a circus performance in an attempt to degrade the party that filed the claim.

And the essential question here is—even if an insurance company wants to "question" an injury claim—why must it be done in a District Court before a jury of "laymen"—many of whom have no knowledge of medicine whatsoever?

Because the powerful, greedy insurance companies have set it up that way. With such a system…they can use all the dramatic, circus acts available to an attorney for putting on court-room trials and trying to convince a jury of "laymen"—as to whether or not someone deserves to be compensated for injuries.

Although the laws that regulate insurance claim procedures state that such cases where there is clear liability and injury—should not be pushed into the Court System—this system has been repeatedly abused by most of the major insurance companies, such as State Farm, All State, Geico and others.

Yet, the benefits and coverage to the consumers and those who make claims is not of much worth. FAR TOO MANY of the insurance policies are never honored whenever there is an accident or sickness.

And worse—injured parties, patients, and consumers have very little protection against these "insurance dictators"!!

Most of the big companies that we hear about in the TV commercials are now and have been using "bad faith" actions in order to evade payment of claims for injuries, damages, medical bills—etc. They simply do not pay the claim and then use the Courts, crooked IME doctors, slander and other acts of subtle terrorism to fight off anyone who makes a claim.

The major insurance companies in the USA have been unfairly and illegally failing to pay legitimate claims. Many of them engage in altering or manipulating medical reviews and reports. Some of these big insurance companies like STATE FARM and GEICO have been investigated and found to be dealing in all sorts of unethical practices, such as manipulating medical reports and/or using used parts to repair cars.

However, the practices continue. Perhaps because there is a lot of money being made by attorneys, insurance companies, politicians and other who permit injured and sick people to be victimized—regardless of who gets hurt or how many lives are ruined.

And attorneys are not solving the problems. Many attorneys are faced with a nearly impossible fight against these insurance monsters. Many so-called injury attorneys are not qualified to fight the monsters. And some of them are just plain corrupt. Some injury attorneys are only interested in cases that may pay them "big bucks"—and will not help the person who has a case worth maybe only $200,000. or less. Attorneys may not openly state this—but many of them will not even take a case that they deem to not be worth more than $100,000. So— people who suffer injuries that "heal up"—may be left without any legal help.

In essence—insurance companies have nearly turned medical injury problems, claims for damages, health care (and related) into nothing more that a cruel and vicious MONEY GAME… a major scam on the American public.

FYI—BELOW THERE IS A SUMMARY OF A STORY OF STATE FARM'S TERRIBLE ILLEGAL ACTIONS AGAINST AN INJURED BLACK AMERICAN WOMAN. Her story is typical and representative of what has been done to many other injured people of all races, ages, and background.

THE FOLLOWING STORY IS TRUE.... taken from an Affidavit:

**WITNESS STATEMENT:*

"I know first-hand that STATE FARM INSURANCE practices absolutely crooked, illegal, fraudulent, and devious acts against people who file claims against them.....

THE FOLLOWING IS A SUMMARY OF THE 3-RING CIRCUS AND CLOWN ACT WHICH STATE FARM INSURANCE PERFORMED FOR US——

My wonderful mother *(who has been a teacher and business trainer for many years)* was struck by a careless driver in Las Vegas while she was walking in a crosswalk. The driver had violated his red light and the white lines for the crosswalk. His truck hit her and thrust her on her head first. She was taken from the scene of the accident by an ambulance. The medic reported that upon their arrival, they found her lying on the ground. She suffered serious injuries to her head, neck, spinal column, arm and shoulder.

She was treated with all types of medications, massage, traction, and other therapies—because of the nature of the severity of the soft tissue damage. State Farm Insurance was the insurance for the driver who had broken the law. He struck her inside the crosswalk with a large Dodge Ram truck. She had the green light and the driver had the red light. The driver was not paying attention while entering the intersection and did strike her with his big truck.

From the very beginning STATE FARM INSURANCE began a campaign against her trying to degrade, discredit and harm my mother. These acts were not only based upon State Farm's normal unethical and "bad faith" policies to evade payment of claims—but were in fact nothing more than a RACIAL ATTACK upon my African-American mother. There were several incidents and actions that show that "race" was used as the main criteria in how this case was handled. And there are numerous other cases where Black people who were injured and filed a claim have been absolutely mis-treated by State Farm.

Before this accident, she was very healthy, athletic and rode her bike for miles every week. After that accident she could not ride her bike at all and she suffers continually and must have on-going therapy...due to the nature of injuries to her nerves, ligaments, tendons, muscles and other tissue. She did receive a lot of treatments and therapy which helped her—but the injuries were very debilitating.

My younger brother and I had to take care of my mother while she suffered in great pain from a head injury, injury to her spinal column, nerves, ligaments, tendons and muscles. She had lots of problems for years and never has been totally relieved of her chronic pain caused by injury to her spinal column. She limps and gets tired very easily—even now after all this time after the accident. She has never been the same since the date of that accident in 1997.

Although State Farm was fully aware of the driver's negligence, and fully aware that the driver had admitted his violation of the red light and traffic violation of hitting a pedestrian in the crosswalk—fully aware that my mother was severely injured from that date in Nov. 1997,—they proceeded to attempt to distort, twist, cover-up and lie about the case—just to keep from compensating this person of color for her injuries. STATE FARM hired an unethical attorney who went above and beyond the call of duty to attack my mother, to slander her, and to illegally evade payment or any kind of compensation.

State Farm did indulge in all types of illegal, crooked, and under-handed things to keep from compensating my mother's doctors and to pay her for her suffering. They have lied, distorted facts, falsified an IME report, violated a COURT ORDER, violated Court Procedures, committed acts of illegal discrimination, and covered up evidence…and much worse!

The insurance adjusters, the attorneys and every other person involved that did not possess a medical license were trying to "diagnose" my mother—and to contradict the highly qualified doctors who did help her and treat her. Contrary to anything that any of the treating doctors and therapists wrote in their reports—State Farm had incompetent attorneys and adjusters trying to make their own fraudulent diagnoses…and did write horrible, threatening and illegal letters to my mother saying in effect—*"they see no value in injuries to her head, spinal column, nerves, tendons & ligaments—that caused her to limp, have chronic full body pain and be disabled for more than 4 years…."*

State Farm paid a crooked IME doctor to *"examine her"* and write a FRAUDULENT MEDICAL REPORT….in which he lied—even though at least a dozen other doctors, specialists and therapists did verify that she suffered from serious, debilitating injuries. He did not fully or appropriately examine her at all. Dr. Oliveri was this IME and he probably already had his fraudulent report written before she ever went to him. You see, State Farm has also been involved in fabricating medical reports.

And in this case—the IME simply lied and tried to claim that my mother's injuries were caused by "old trauma." Dr. Oliveri was acting in collusion with State Farm to help the evade payment of the injury claim. My mother had been seriously injured and these White Males sat in their fancy offices and prepared phoney paper-work and reports, hired crooked lawyers and slandered my mother—JUST TO KEEP FROM COMPENSATING HER DOCTORS and paying for her DISABILITY.

Dr. Oliveri performed an "exam" that was totally superficial and could not assess whether my mother had the flu, cancer, or a broken rib. Then he wrote a "report"—that was not based upon any objective testing (such as X-rays or scans). He stated that her pain was caused by "old injuries." HE IS A LIAR. I should know since I have lived with her for over 20 years. And this IME did not have any other medical reports that indicated that there were ever any old injuries to my mother's spinal column or muscles (etc.) Had she been injured like this previously—she would have already accumulated extensive medical bills—and been disabled.

I happen to know that there never were any types of injuries to her spinal column—NO CONCUSSIONS, NO SEVERE MUSCLE SPRAINS, NO FULL BODY CHRONIC PAIN——nothing like this ever before in my mother's history. It was all a "set up" by State Farm's adjusters who told this IME what to write.

This IME doctor regularly works for State Farm and his job is to invent fraudulent medical reports in order to help the insurance company evade paying claims. State Farm has spent a lot of time and money hiring a crooked attorney—who violated nearly every law on the books in order to try to harm my injured mother and not pay her doctors.

Since I am a direct witness to everything—I can verify that STATE FARM and their reps/attorneys did in fact deal in lies, corruption, fraud, harassment, stalking and other illegal actions against my mother…without one bit of evidence in their defense.

Because we know that my mother was illegally discriminated against, and because we have met other Black people who had similar experiences with State Farm——my brother and I are convinced that these acts were based upon "illegal racial discrimination" and " white racism"—that we were treated so badly because we are NOT-WHITE PEOPLE—

and we are aware of other minority people who have been discriminated against by State Farm Insurance Co. We know of at least 3 other cases where Black women were badly injured— State Farm was liable—and State Farm used every underhanded, illegal, dirty trick in the book to keep from compensating these accident victims—including racial discrimination.

One Black woman was struck by a careless driver and seriously injured. The driver of the truck was a white man. State Farm fought this woman for 6 years—without one ounce of evidence in their behalf. After 6 years—this weary old woman finally settled for far less than the case was worth. We also know of another Black woman who was hit from behind and injured— by a white driver in Texas. She was dragged thru considerable dirt, muck and mire by State Farm—taken to a Court room before an all-white jury and slandered by State Farm Insurance and their attorneys. She was in the U.S. Air Force—and State Farm slandered this woman in court to a level of out-right devilishment. The attorneys for State Farm used "race" as an issue and made constant implications to the white jury that this Black woman was trying to cheat them....even though white doctors testified that she was really injured.

Yes, in addition to State Farm's normal "bad faith actions"— —we also believe that State Farm went above and beyond the call of duty to try to evade payment of this claim because they use racist policies and we are African- Americans (black people). We have heard a lot of "nightmare" stories from other people of color who have been mis-treated by STATE FARM INSURANCE CO.

It is widely known that State Farm mis-treats millions of people for any reason they want to choose for the occasion. If you are Black—that is a good reason for State Farm Insurance to lie on you and try to get you in front of a racist all-white jury in order to stage a drama before these unsuspecting jurors.

Now, Nevada is not the most liberal state or the most "honest" either—and it is the perfect place for State Farm to practice "bad faith." All of the people who attacked my mother were WHITE MALES from the red-neck city of Las Vegas, NV. In fact, Las Vegas in well known for its bad past and history of being known as *"The Mississippi of the West."*

Believe me…State Farm has perfected these "bad faith actions" to a near-SCIENCE. They utilize FORMULAS in order to fight any case they so choose to not pay. State Farm has been exposed in TV documentaries to be guilty of changing or manipulating medical reports, of lying, using fraud, and of other illegal actions.

One of their formulas against minority people IS TO TAKE THESE CASES TO COURT AND TRY TO IMPRESS THE MOSTLY WHITE JURY THAT THE INJURED PARTY IS OF LOW CHARACTER—is exploiting negative stereotypes of non-White people——to falsely claim that these peope are "*exaggerating their injuries*"—in order to "not work"—— preying upon old racist stereotypes of "*lazy blacks*"—and "*black people who steal.*"

STATE FARM will do nearly anything—legal or not—to evade paying a claim.

THIS MAY ALL SOUND UNBELIEVABLE—but it is a true story!!

SOUND UNBELIEVABLE???——Ask your own doctor… LET YOUR OWN HEALTH CARE PROVIDERS— (Therapists, Chiropractors, Physicians, etc.)… TELL YOU ABOUT THEIR OWN HORROR STORIES OF TRYING TO COLLECT PAYMENT FROM INSURANCE COMPANIES.

My mother and her legal assistants sent a long, detailed written report of all of this FRAUD to the U.S. Senate, Federal Trade Commission, Insurance Commission, Civil Rights Commission, and the Nevada Legislature and requested a FORMAL INVESTIGATION of State Farm Insurance Co. So far these politicians, Insurance Commissions, and Civil Rights agencies have been silent. My mother still continues to suffer from these injuries and has been declared disabled.

All of State Farm's actions in this case alone should put the adjusters, attorneys and staff in prison for a long time. If a regular citizen committed ONE of these actions….s/he would be in prison for it. However, our legislators, judges, insurance commissioners, senators, etc. seem to have buried their heads in the sand when it comes to this high-level fraud and corruption that is going on with the insurance industry.

I say to anyone who owns insurance from State Farm Insurance to get rid of it!! They are corrupt and will harm anyone and everyone that they can—just to get rich.

This present SYSTEM is designed to pay insurance attorneys, adjusters, private investigators and crooked doctors—while simultaneously refusing to pay the injured party and doctors, clinics, and therapists who treated the injured party.

I am shocked that the government allows them to continue to do business. But then again—I figure that someone at the top is benefitting financially from mis-treating injured people and allowing these insurance companies to get away with these acts of terrorism.

Submitted by Mr. M. Price of Las Vegas, NV
E-mail= spiritualnews@hotmail.com

****

EXPLANATION:

Major insurance companies are simply refusing to pay legitimate claims. This widespread social problem is that of "bad faith insurance companies." Thousands and millions of Americans have been suffering at the hands of crooked and unethical insurance companies…who utilize everything from fraud, dirty tricks, crooked IME doctors and much worse—in order to avoid paying claims for damages and injuries. Insurance companies require huge payment for their policies and services, but they arbitrarily refuse to pay for any claim that they see fit…for no legitimate reason.

Anyone who drives a car is required by law to purchase vehicle insurance. If someone drives without insurance—it becomes another case for the courts. Employers are expected to provide medical coverage for their workers. And yet—the insurance giants operate virtually unsupervised.

Attorneys and insurance adjusters are practicing medicine without a license, changing medical reports, using fraudulent IME doctors….calling highly educated doctors into question….and much worse—in order to keep from compensating and injured party or from paying for other losses.

The Courts have often ruled against many of these crooked insurance companies—but the essential question is WHY is the system so pathetic that millions of people have to fight these insurance companies in Court in the first place???In fact, the Courts and attorneys are making almost as much money as the Insurance companies.

Our law-makers, politicians, governors, senators, etc. have established a system that works for the benefit of insurance companies, but offers the owners of policies and victims of accidents little more than the chance to hunt for a "qualified attorney" and to litigate cases for years against unscrupulous, callous insurance companies who simply refuse to pay legitimate claims.

If you are concerned about the state of our world, then you must be concerned about the horrible tactics being employed by greedy insurance companies.

There are few protections for the consumer or injured patients who are being mis-treated daily by these "goliaths."

READ MORE ABOUT THIS ISSUE OF BAD FAITH AT THIS WEB-SITE:

http://www.badfaithinsurance.org

ACTUAL "bad faith" STORIES:

And to receive a copy of actual complaints, horror stories, and other cases of insurance company fraud—and/or to find out about how you can have possible have your "bad faith story" published——contact the author & publisher of this book.

To get more details about a book to be published on this issue, visit this website:

http://mypages.blackvoices.com/museum

WHO PROTECTS THE CONSUMERS AGAINST THESE INSURANCE MONSTERS—WHO HELPS THE INJURED PARTIES, AND THE PEOPLE WHO MAKE CLAIMS for damages, pain & suffering, etc. ??

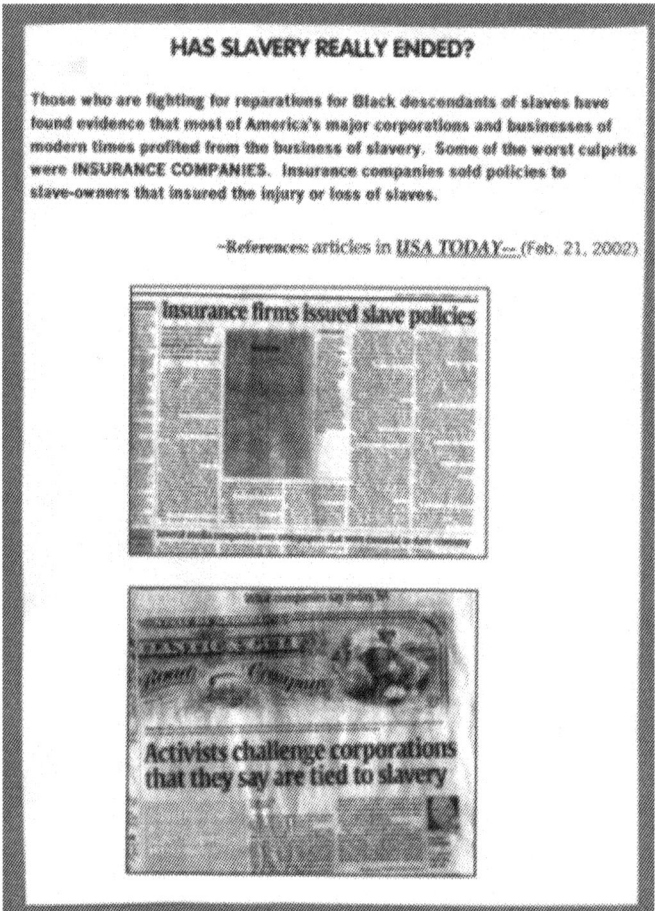

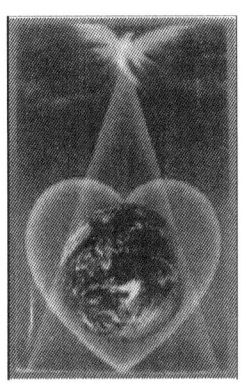

"SPIRITUAL BLESSINGS"—by Melvia Miller

A man questioned whether or not a God of the Universe really exists. Whenever people mentioned "God"—this man claimed that he could not see, feel, hear, or taste this God.

The man whispered, *"God, speak to me"*

And a meadowlark sang.

"God—if you really exist—let me see or hear or smell you…"—this man continued to beg for answers to this pressing question—as he stood in his own beautiful garden where he grew tomatoes, onions, corn, greens, and lettuce every year.

But the man did not see any significance to these wonderous things.

So the man yelled *"God, speak to me"*

And the thunder & lightning rolled across the sky.

But the man did not listen.

The man looked around and said, *"God, let me see you."*

And a star shined brightly. But the man did not see anything significant in the vast skies.

And, the man shouted, *"God, show me a miracle"*—

And a new baby was born to him and his wife ….but the man did not see any meaning in this event.

So, the man cried out in despair,——

"Touch me, God, and let me know you are here"—

Whereupon, God reached down and touched the man.

But the man brushed the butterfly away and walked on.

The man cried *"God, I need your help"*…and an e-mail arrived reaching out with good news, a business opportunity, and encouragement.

But the man deleted it and continued whining and crying….

After many weeks of his blind complaining and doubting—this man got in his Toyota sports car, drove up the highway to the mountains and sat there to just think this problem over…. this man stood on top of a mountain over-looking the fabulous ocean, and begged—
—*"God—if you are there—let me see you."*

Then the man looked up toward the sky and he saw a strange UFO dart past. But he continued to whine and beg.

****

***MORAL OF THIS STORY=

Don't miss out on a blessing because it isn't packaged the way that you expect. The good news is that you are loved. The universe is abundant in all that is good, pure, beautiful and strong.

RECOMMENDED WEBSITES:

Government Grants: find out how you can get money to go to school, for your business or for writing a book—and much more!

www.freegovmoney.net

MEDLINE: Health Information selected by the Nat. Library of Medicine:

www.medlineplus.gov

American Dietetic Association= *Link nutrition and health*
www.eatright.org

American Botanical Council: Learn more about herbs—
www.herbalgram.org

Start your own home-based publishing business!
    Visit:
www.maxpages.com/freepress

FREE ON-LINE BUSINESS OPPORTUNITY NEWSLETTER:

www.maxpages.com/seminar/newsletter

You could win $1,000 by knowing a lot about history....

Visit the TRUE HISTORY MUSEUM:

http://mypages.blackvoices.com/truehistory

ARE YOU LOOKING FOR WAYS TO BECOME
HEALTHIER & WEALTHIER?
FIND OUT MORE ABOUT THE WONDERFUL
HERBAL PRODUCTS

http://mypages.blackvoices.com/greatspirit

=======================================

EARN WHILE YOU LEARN—
    YOU CAN GET A VALUABLE CERTIFICATE OF ACHIEVEMENT
BY COMPLETING THE
"Workshop on the Web"

    http://www.maxpages.com/seminar
=======================================

RECOMMENDED BOOKS:

* As a Man Thinketh—by James Allen

* *African American Inventors—by P. & J. McKissack*

* *African Americans and the Revolutionary War—by Judith Harper*

* *Back To Eden—by Jethro Kloss*

* *Before the Mayflower————by Lerone Bennett*

* *BREAKING THE CHAINS OF PSYCHOLOGICAL SLAVERY—by Dr.*
Naim Akbar

* *Eat for Your Blood Type—by Dr. Peter J. D'Adamo*

* *HEALING THE SHAME THAT BINDS YOU—*
by John Bradshaw

* *How Europe Underdeveloped Africa—*
by Dr. Walter Rodney

* HOW TO WIN FRIENDS AND INFLUENCE PEOPLE…. By Dale
Carnegie

* "I'm OK—You're OK"—by Dr. Thomas A. Harris

* *Mis-Education of the Negro*————*by Dr. Carter Woodson*

* "Negative Criticism" by Sidney Simon

* *One Hundred Thousand Years of Man's Unknown History*—by Robert Charroux

* *"Racial Healing"*—by Harlon Dulton

* *"Self-Parenting Workbook"* ......
(Windows to Your Inner Child)—by—Dr. P. Gorman & P. Diaz

* *They Came Before Columbus*—by I.V. Sertima

* *"THE HEALING PATH" (A Soul Approach to Illness)*
By M. Barasch

* *Roots*—by Alex Haley

* *The Destruction of Black Civilization*—by Chancellor Williams

* *The Herb Bible*—by Dr. Earl Mindell

* *The Middle Passage*—by Dr. John Henrik Clarke

* *The Mysterious Past*—by Robert Charroux

EDUCATIONAL GAMES

Activities, Exercises and Games make learning more fun and effective. This section on games is presented to enhance studying and learning about the subjects presented in this book.

These exercises and games can be adapted to nearly any subject—such as: Nutrition, Black History, Spanish, etc.

HUNT -A -RHYME GAME

<u>Purpose</u>: To help develop "phonics"
Skills in sounds of words.

<u>Materials needed</u>: At least 60 cards with
Words printed on them. There
must be at least one other word
that sounds like (rhymes with)
each word. Use words from a
story participants have read.

Examples: Van — - Man — Ran
Game — - Name——Shame
Head——Said——Red

<u>How To Play:</u> Spread the cards out on a table
with words showing. Select one.
*Give each player one chance to pick another
word that rhymes with the one selected.

*If the player answers *incorrectly*,
S/he loses one turn.
*If the player answers *correctly*,
the player can continue to
Match rhyming words until
s/he misses.

****
<u>Winner:</u>   Whoever collects the most cards with
Rhyming words on them **WINS**.
****

Prizes can be awarded.

| LOOK |

| BOOK |

| TOOK |

ROCK SCHOOL:

LEARNING GOALS & OBJECTIVES:
    To practice answering questions with facts, and
    to learn more about History.

MATERIALS NEEDED TO PARTICIPATE IN THIS ACTIVITY:

** This game should be played on a set of bleachers or steps.

**A list of at least 50 questions/answers on the facts & heroes
        of Black History.

    ...Example- QUESTION: What is the name of the famous
            Black Basketball team that began in 1927
            and won more than 8,000 victories?

            ANSWER: "The Harlem Globetrotters."

How To Play: * One participant serves as *"teacher."*

* The steps are considered to be "grade levels."
    Bottom step is *Kindergarten*, next step is
    First grade.....and on up.
    The top step is *"Graduation."*
* Participants start at *Kindergarten* level by sitting there.

*The teacher hides a stone or rock *in one hand*
    behind his/her back...then shows both fists to
    each student one at a time. That student must
    guess which fist is hiding the stone. If the student
    chooses correctly, the student gets to answer a question
    that the teacher selects from the list. If the student
    answers correctly, he/she moves up to sit on the next
    Higher step. Every player moves up until someone wins.*
        *""If the student does not guess
        correctly either question, he/she
        stays on the same step (loses a turn)
        until he/she gets the correct answers.*

* THE *WINNER* is the student who reaches the top step first.

fitness

herbs

hormones

minerals

nutrition

organic

protein

vitality

vitamins

wellness

WORD DEFINITION CHAIN

<u>Objective:</u> To have fun learning
          the correct definitions of words.

Materials Needed:
* Strips of colored paper (approx. 2" wide
    And 5" long) to be used to paste together
    a paper chain.
* Glue stick (or paste).
* Dictionary (or flash cards).

How to Play:
    Prepare a list of words to be used in
The game on cards. Put the new vocabulary
word on one side, with its meaning on the
opposite side. Or words can be listed on
a sheet with the *meanings* on another sheet.

Having a minimum of 3 players makes this game fun.
One player serves as the "caller" and chooses the word
to be defined from the list.

Players go in turn--- Each player tries to give the correct
definition of the word next on the list. If a player
gives the wrong definition, s/he loses one turn and
cannot add any links to the chain.
    Whenever a player gives the correct definition,
s/he gets to make one link in his/her paper chain,
using a paper strip and gluing it onto the rest of
the chain. The player who makes the longest chain, *WINS.*

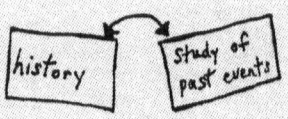

FOR EXAMPLE---

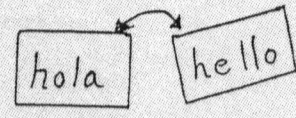

THE HOLISTIC REMEDY MATCH GAME

INSTRUCTIONS: Match the name of the Herb (nutrient)
             with its correct benefit...by drawing a line
             across to each matching set.

HERB/NUTRIENT: BENEFIT:

* Ginseng   * Alleviates depression &
                                   nervous ailments.

* Black Cohosh   * Good anti-biotic against
                                   colds and flu.

* Witch Hazel   * Old remedy for calming
                                   colic, convulsions, PMS.

*Goldenseal   * Stimulates energy.
                                   Prevents many diseases...

*Catnip   * Good for female hormone
                                   ...estrogen replacement.

*St. john's Wort   * Stimulates thyroid,
                                   helps weight loss.

* L-Carnitine   *Fights cancerus tumors

* MSM   * Repairs & rebuilds tissue.
                                   alleviates aches & pains.
                                   (Organic Sulfur)

*Kelp   * Stops diarrhea, hemorrhaging;
                                   & inflammation; heals bed sores

* Emu Oil   * Amino acid good for heart,
                                   lowers blood pressure.

* Essiac Tea---   * Comes from a rare bird....
                                   alleviates arthritis,
                                   skin problems, and more.

More
ACTIVITIES, EXERCISES, and GAMES

AVAILABLE.....

This unique collection of stories, fables, and articles on topics such as: HEALTH, WEALTH, PROSPERITY, RACIAL HARMONY, CULTURAL DIVERSITY——

.....Also comes with a separate booklet of....EXERCISES, GAMES AND ACTIVITIES TO HELP MAKE LEARNING MORE FUN AND EFFECTIVE.

A WORKBOOK is available separately, which is filled with educational exercises, games and activities—

Please contact MOTHERSHIP PUBLICATIONS to get more details and order forms.

E-Mail= culturaldiversity@hotmail.com

WHAT OUR READERS SAY:

"Melvia's books are very useful, excellent, and inspiring."

—from Dr. Carmela Corallo, **(Director of Infinite Winds Counseling Center*—of Encinitas, CA)

∗∗

"Melvia Miller writes an excellent brand of poetry."

~ Max Robinson, (ABC—TV News anchorman)

∗∗∗∗∗∗

"Melvia Miller brings to her work a solid background as an educator and a member of a minority group, which make her books of a true multi-cultural perspective. We thank Melvia for her wonderful contributions."

…from Dr. Penny Ralston, *Dean—Florida State Univ.*

∗∗∗∗∗∗∗∗∗∗∗∗∗∗∗∗∗∗∗∗∗∗∗∗∗∗∗∗∗∗∗∗∗∗∗∗∗∗

"Melvia Miller's book…is a fun and filled with activities and exercises to make learning about health fun. We recommend that you read this book—not once—but twice and even thrice. It is full of important information."

~ by "The Mooney Twins"—Dwayne Mooney
(aka: *The Conscious Comedy Duo)* of Los Angeles, CA

****

"I am indeed impressed with Melvia's books. I look forward to reading more from her."

—from Dr. Gloria Murray, *Professor—Indiana Univ.—*
Louisville,KY

****

"I commend Melvia Miller on her ingenuity and creativity in writing these books. Her stories and articles are very well written. She has created some of the most interesting and fun materials I have ever seen on this subject."

~ Ms. Joan Cox, Distinctive Arts Publishing
"Write-A-Book-Class, INC."—(Las Vegas, NV)
****

"Melvia's stories are REAL AND WONDERFUL... She does a good job in illustrating how the tradition "medical" therapies and the "alternative holistic therapies" each have a place in helping us to improve our health. She brings out many real and earthy concepts which help us to become more aware. Awareness can help us heal."

—by Ms. Donna Dowdell, R.N.—*(*Director of Holistic Temple of Las Vegas, NV)*

✳✳✳

"Melvia has a unique way of making us laugh at ourselves in order to grow and change. This author's fables contain a lot of symbolism and humor that sheds light on the social problems and bring home the points that she is making with potency."

~By Ms. Debra Williams—*Behavioral Health Specialist;*
East Chicago, IN

✳✳✳✳✳✳✳✳✳✳✳✳✳✳✳✳✳✳✳✳

"Melvia Miller has made learning history and cultural subjects enjoyable and interesting. Her workshops are creative, interactive and educational. I hope she continues to write these fantastic books on cultural diversity and Black History."

—~Ms. Anke McKiernan *(Marketing Consultant of Vista,CA)*

This is another book from the "Super Sistah" series collection....of healing words.

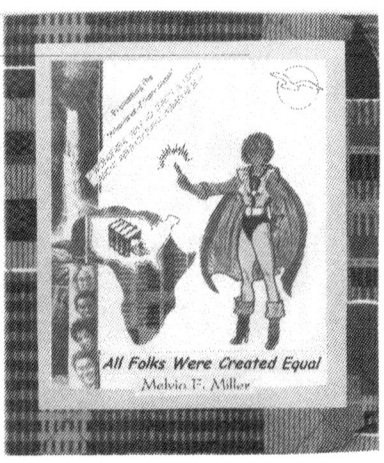

HAVE A MILLION DOLLAR DAY—

A manual and workbook to help you increase your income and improve your life.

*Learn to write a business plan
* Inc. and Grow Rich

LEARN SOURCES TO GET PRODUCTS SUCH AS—

Motivational & spiritual books & information
Herbal & natural health products
Multi-cultural books, videos, and CDs
Cultural art & souvenirs
Black History posters & workbooks
Urban gear and hip-hop (style) clothing
Afro-centric, ethnic-style clothing

African Imports
Oriental and Native American arts & crafts
Educational products

FOR MORE DETAILS ON HOW TO GET A CATALOG, CONTACT
US BY E-MAIL:

culturaldiversity@hotmail.com

Created, compiled and composed by *Diversity Promotions Co.*

ABOUT THE AUTHOR:

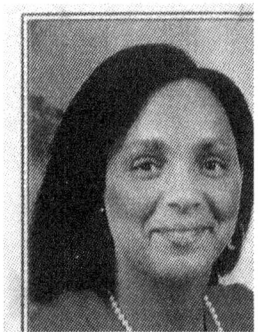

Award-winning author Melvia F. Miller

Melvia Miller has been active in the professional arena of instructional design, consulting, training and preparation of business manuals. Melvia has a special talent for creating effective and fun learning materials, and she is an expert in the area of designing educational materials for teaching cultural diversity and Black History.

She has received many honors and awards, fellowships, and scholarships, including having been named to *"Who's Who in American Universities & Colleges."* and the *"Young Professional Woman of the Year"*—by NANBPW.

Melvia Miller grew up in Muncie, IN—and has also written a series of books concerning the African-American experiences in that town and in the USA.

Melvia is the author of several other books, manuals, and workbooks.

Melvia is a graduate of the University of Michigan and Ball State University. She holds several degrees from other programs and institutes as well.

She is the mother of 2 sons: Malik & Mikal